PRINCIPLES OF ACUTE CARE NURSING

PRINCIPLES OF ACUTE CARE NURSING

SARAH MCGLOIN
ALICE SKULL

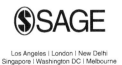

Los Angeles | London | New Delhi
Singapore | Washington DC | Melbourne

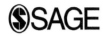

Los Angeles | London | New Delhi
Singapore | Washington DC | Melbourne

SAGE Publications Ltd
1 Oliver's Yard
55 City Road
London EC1Y 1SP

SAGE Publications Inc.
2455 Teller Road
Thousand Oaks, California 91320

SAGE Publications India Pvt Ltd
B 1/I 1 Mohan Cooperative Industrial Area
Mathura Road
New Delhi 110 044

SAGE Publications Asia-Pacific Pte Ltd
3 Church Street
#10-04 Samsung Hub
Singapore 049483

Editor: Alex Clabburn
Assistant editor: Ruth Lilly
Production editor: Sarah Cooke
Copyeditor: Christine Bitten
Proofreader: Salia Nessa
Indexer: Judith Lavender
Cover design: Sheila Tong
Typeset by: C&M Digitals (P) Ltd, Chennai, India

© Sarah McGloin and Alice Skull 2022

Apart from any fair dealing for the purposes of research, private study, or criticism or review, as permitted under the Copyright, Designs and Patents Act, 1988, this publication may not be reproduced, stored or transmitted in any form, or by any means, without the prior permission in writing of the publisher, or in the case of reprographic reproduction, in accordance with the terms of licences issued by the Copyright Licensing Agency. Enquiries concerning reproduction outside those terms should be sent to the publisher.

Library of Congress Control Number: 2022935598

British Library Cataloguing in Publication data

A catalogue record for this book is available from the British Library.

ISBN 978-1-5264-2418-1
ISBN 978-1-5264-2419-8 (pbk)

DEDICATION

This is in recognition to all the healthcare workers who have demon–strated such resilience and commitment to caring for so many, often in clinical settings that are new and different to them, throughout the COVID-19 pandemic.

TABLE OF CONTENTS

ABOUT THE AUTHOR

Alice Skull MSc Interprofessional Practice Health and Social Care, BSc (Hons) Health Studies, DipHE Registered Nurse Adult, PGDip Learning & Teaching is a Senior Lecturer in Adult Nursing and Course Leader for the Registered Nurse adult apprenticeship at Anglia Ruskin University (ARU) and has over 17 years' experience in the practice, theory and education at postgraduate and undergraduate level. Alice began her nursing career in 1996, working in cardiac care and medical nursing. This interest in cardiac nursing has continued through leadership of the post registration cardiac care module, along with development of a wide range of knowledge and experience in acute care. Alice is particularly interested in workforce development through the nursing apprenticeship route and pastoral care of nursing students.

Sarah McGloin PhD RN SFHEA worked for a number of years on a regional neurosurgical, burns and general critical care unit, after which she moved into nurse education where she held a number of roles including Course lead for Critical Care and Advanced Clinical Practice. During this time, she completed her PhD which explored critically ill patients' reconstructive memories of critical care and nurses' understanding and response to these. Sarah is now the Head of Grants and Impact at the RCN Foundation which is an independent nursing charity which supports all nurses, midwives and healthcare support workers through its grant-making activities.

1

CARE OF THE ACUTELY ILL ADULT

ALICE SKULL

Chapter learning outcomes

By the end of this chapter you will be able to:

1. Discuss the context of using a systematic approach to assessing and monitoring care.
2. Identify the components of an ABCDE approach.
3. Examine the factors to be included in assessment using an ABCDE approach.
4. Discuss the importance of providing timely and appropriate management.
5. Demonstrate awareness of the tools that can assist timely recognition and response to deterioration such as National Early Warning Scoring (NEWS2), ACVPU, Critical Care Outreach Teams, SBAR.
6. Recognise the importance of situational awareness and why patient safety is central to all care decisions.

Key words

- ABCDE Resuscitation Council UK
- NEWS2 Royal College of Physicians
- ACVPU
- Critical Care Outreach
- SBAR
- Situational awareness
- Patient safety
- Person-centred care

The chapter will outline the ABCDE approach to assessing the acutely ill adult. To assist this, the key national drivers relating to acute care practice will be introduced. The context and background to contemporary acute care practice will also be discussed. Communication, NEWS2 and SBAR will be included.

At the point of registration, the registered nurse must be able to demonstrate the knowledge and ability to respond proactively and promptly to signs of deterioration or distress in mental, physical, cognitive and behavioural health, and use this knowledge to make sound clinical decisions (NMC, 2018).

Using a systematic approach to assessment and care of the acutely ill adult is not a new phenomenon. The National Patient Safety Agency's (NPSA) – now part of NHS England - report in 2007 identified that out of 425 reported deaths in acute care, 64 were related to patient deterioration not being recognised or acted upon (15%). Learning from these serious incidents and examples of suboptimal care contributed to the focus on tools to aid recognition and timely intervention for patients at risk of clinical deterioration. A search of a reliable nursing database such as Cumulative Index to Nursing and Allied Health Literature (CINAHL) now identifies thousands of articles focused on this topic.

At the end of the last century, McQuillan et al. (1998), in a confidential inquiry, examined the prevalence, nature, causes and consequences of suboptimal care, identifying that the management of airway, breathing, circulation and oxygen therapy and monitoring in severely ill patients may frequently be suboptimal. The term *suboptimal* is subjective and reliant on the interpretation of those retrospectively assessing risk but is based on meaning that care is below an optimal standard, which may be caused by organisational failure, a lack of knowledge and failure to appreciate the urgency of the situation. They proposed that the structure and process of acute care required major re-evaluation and debate. This evaluation has been ongoing and in 2016 NHS Improvement reported that of the death and severe harm incidents reported in acute hospitals, 7% related to a failure to recognise or act on deterioration.

The National Institute for Health and Care Excellence (NICE) (2007) guidance relating to acutely ill adults in hospital focuses on the measurement and recording of a set of physiological observations linked to a 'track and trigger' system. Track and trigger means a process must be in place to identify (track) patients who are deteriorating and to take action (trigger) based on these findings. NICE (2007) emphasises the importance of a full clinical assessment, training, and that patient safety is best ensured when there are clear response strategies in place.

NEWS2 (Royal College of Physicians, 2017) is the latest version of the National Early Warning Score (NEWS), first produced in 2012 and updated in December 2017, which advocates a system to standardise the assessment and response to acute illness. It has been widely adopted in England due to its endorsement from NHS England and NHS Improvement. NEWS2 is based on measurement of six physiological parameters:

1. Respiration rate
2. Oxygen saturation
3. Systolic blood pressure
4. Pulse rate
5. Level of consciousness or new confusion
6. Temperature

A score is allocated to each parameter as it is recorded, and the higher the score the more abnormal the result (range 0–3). The score is then aggregated and uplifted by two points for people requiring supplemental oxygen to maintain their recommended oxygen saturation. It should be noted that the trigger ranges displayed on the NEWS2 chart (see Figure 1.1) are not entirely consistent with normal physiological ranges, for example NEWS2 does not trigger for systolic blood pressure between 111 mmHg and 219 mmHg although these would be defined as hypertensive (NICE, 2019). Similarly, the influence of chronic disease such as Chronic Obstructive Pulmonary Disease (COPD) and chronic heart failure also need to be factored in as, for example, patients with COPD are likely to have an elevated heart rate, increased respiratory rate and decreased oxygen saturations during sub optimal (RCP) periods of health.

Physiological parameter	Score						
	3	2	1	0	1	2	3
Respiration rate (per minute)	≤8		9–11	12–20		21–24	≥25
SpO$_2$ Scale 1 (%)	≤91	92–93	94–95	≥96			
SpO$_2$ Scale 2 (%)	≤83	84–85	86–87	88–92 ≥93 on air	93–94 on oxygen	95–96 on oxygen	≥97 on oxygen
Air or oxygen?		Oxygen		Air			
Systolic blood pressure (mmHg)	≤90	91–100	101–110	111–219			≥220
Pulse (per minute)	≤40		41–50	51–90	91–110	111–130	≥131
Consciousness				Alert			CVPU
Temperature (°C)	≤35.0		35.1–36.0	36.1–38.0	38.1–39.0	≥39.1	

Figure 1.1   The NEWS scoring system Chart 1

Source: Reproduced from Royal College of Physicians (2017). *National Early Warning Score (NEWS) 2: Standardising the assessment of acute-illness severity in the NHS.* Updated report of a working party. London: RCP.

Activity 1.1

Access https://news.ocbmedia.com/ and complete the NEWS2 e-learning tool.

Place the certificate in your portfolio and write a reflective piece identifying what you have learnt. This could be used for evidence of continuing professional development and professional body revalidation.

Consider what non-technical skills the nurse will require to effectively assess a patient.

Having tracked a patient's observations, NEWS2 outlines a series of response triggers and frequency of monitoring required (see Figure 1.2). Electronic systems will aggregate the score and some will initiate this clinical response electronically alerting the appropriate clinician to review the patient.

NEW score	Frequency of monitoring	Clinical response
0	Minimum 12 hourly	• Continue routine NEWS monitoring
Total 1–4	Minimum 4–6 hourly	• Inform registered nurse, who must assess the patient • Registered nurse decides whether increased frequency of monitoring and/or escalation of care is required
3 in single parameter	Minimum 1 hourly	• Registered nurse to inform medical team caring for the patient, who will review and decide whether escalation of care is necessary
Total 5 or more Urgent response threshold	Minimum 1 hourly	• Registered nurse to immediately inform the medical team caring for the patient • Registered nurse to request urgent assessment by a clinician or team with core competencies in the care of acutely ill patients • Provide clinical care in an environment with monitoring facilities
Total 7 or more Emergency response threshold	Continuous monitoring of vital signs	• Registered nurse to immediately inform the medical team caring for the patient – this should be at least at specialist registrar level • Emergency assessment by a team with critical care competencies, including practitioner(s) with advanced airway management skills • Consider transfer of care to a level 2 or 3 clinical care facility, ie higher-dependency unit or Intensive Care Unit (ICU) • Clinical care in an environment with monitoring facilities

Figure 1.2   Clinical response to the NEWS trigger thresholds Chart 4

Source: Reproduced from Royal College of Physicians (2017). *National Early Warning Score (NEWS) 2: Standardising the assessment of acute-illness severity in the NHS.* Updated report of a working party. London: RCP.

It is essential that all healthcare practitioners are able to effectively use a track and trigger system and demonstrate competence in measuring physiological parameters. It is well documented that some parameters are frequently omitted such as respiratory rate and the emphasis within NEWS2 on this may go some way to rectify this. Nurses, however, will use a range of different skills to assess the acutely unwell patient including many non-technical skills ensuring that assessment is both person-centred and holistic. The ABCDE approach enables nurses to perform a holistic and systematic assessment of deteriorating patients (Resuscitation Council UK, 2021). For clarity it is important to understand what the headings in the ABCDE assessment indicate (see Table 1.1).

Table 1.1   ABCDE assessment

Airway	Assessment of the patency of the airway
Breathing	Assessment of breathing
Circulation	Assessment of the circulatory system
Disability	Neurological assessment of consciousness
Exposure	Head to toe examination of the patient

Source: Resuscitation Council UK, 2015.

The underlying principles of an ABCDE approach have been summarised by the Resuscitation Council UK (2021) as follows:.

- Use the Airway, Breathing, Circulation, Disability, Exposure (ABCDE) approach to assess and treat the patient.
- Complete an initial assessment and reassess regularly.
- Treat life-threatening problems before moving to the next part of assessment.
- Assess the effects of treatment.
- Recognise when you will need extra help and call for help early.
- Use all members of the team and communicate effectively.
- The aim of the initial treatment is to keep the patient alive and achieve some clinical improvement.

Before commencing a systematic assessment the healthcare professional should make a rapid risk assessment of the environment, ensuring that they are safe to approach the patient and that any hazards to themselves or the patient are minimised. For example, are there any trailing cables on the floor, a bowl of water at the bedside or objects that could fall onto them? Appropriate hand hygiene should occur and any necessary personal protective equipment applied. A 'Look, Listen and Feel' approach should be used, firstly assessing the patient in general – do they appear unwell, observe their skin colour, body position, look for non-verbal cues that may indicate pain, distress and anxiety. This rapid assessment should move onto 'listen' and if the patient is awake ask, 'How are you?'. If the patient appears unconscious or has collapsed, shake him/her (not too vigorously so as to cause further trauma) and ask, 'Are you alright?'.

Activity 1.2

Reflect on the difference between the two questions asked in a rapid initial assessment:

- How are you?
- Are you alright?

What is the difference and why are different types of questions used?

If the patient responds normally they have a patent airway, are breathing and have brain perfusion. If they only speak in short sentences, the airway may be at risk. Failure of the patient to respond is a clear marker of critical illness. This rapid assessment should take about 30 seconds (Resuscitation Council UK, 2021).

Actions should be taken in line with the practitioner's scope of practice, clinical competency and training. It should not be forgotten that at the centre of this patient assessment is a person whose dignity must be preserved and that employing a compassionate and respectful approach are the hallmarks of a professional practitioner.

Figure 1.3 at the end of the chapter summarises the initial assessment, measurements, actions and rationale using an ABCDE approach.

Activity 1.3

Using a BNF make a list of drugs that could reduce consciousness and identify their antagonist (antidote).

Activity 1.4

Consider how you want patients to feel when they speak to you. The art of 'active listening' is important to demonstrate that you care and you are receiving all the relevant information. Read: Ali, M. (2018) Communication skills 5: Effective listening and observation. *Nursing Times*, 114(4), 56–57 for practical advice to make you a more effective listener.

Reflect on what you have learnt from reading this article in your professional portfolio.

LEVELS OF CARE

In 2000, the Department of Health published its review of critical care services and with it recommendations for classifying the level of care that patients need. It looked at the whole system from the needs of those at risk of deterioration and critical illness, those who have recovered, and the needs of patients during the critical illness itself. The Intensive Care Society (ICS) published *Levels of Critical Care for Adult Patients* in 2009, which aimed to identify those ward patients who may benefit from higher staffing ratios than were available on wards and access to senior clinical decision makers. The Covid-19 pandemic has seen an escalating demand for critical care beds and in 2021 this guidance was updated with some changes to the original levels of care (ICS, 2021). The level of care required is used as part of a risk assessment strategy and a graded response to escalation of deterioration (NICE, 2007). An understanding of the levels of care will aid in decisions about skill mix and staffing in line with NICE (2014), which emphasises locating patients where their clinical needs can be best met.

Table 1.2 identifies the levels of care with clinical examples.

Table 1.2   Definition of levels of care

Level of care	Criteria	Example
Ward Care	<ul><li>Requires hospitalisation</li><li>Needs can be met through normal ward care</li></ul>	Mohammed is admitted for day surgery and will require post-operative monitoring and intravenous therapy
Level 1 Enhanced Care	<ul><li>Patients recently discharged from a higher level of care</li><li>Patients in need of additional monitoring/clinical interventions, input or advice</li><li>Patients requiring critical care outreach service support</li><li>Patients who would benefit from Enhanced Perioperative Care</li></ul>	Rhonda has been discharged from the high dependency unit where she received respiratory support following surgery. She is receiving continuous oxygen therapy and requires a minimum of four-hourly observations. Other examples include: <ul><li>Fluid resuscitation</li><li>Epidural analgesia in use</li><li>Parenteral nutrition</li><li>Central venous catheter, tracheostomy, chest drain</li><li>Minimum four-hourly GCS</li><li>Continuous insulin infusion</li><li>Established intermittent renal support</li><li>Aggregate score 5–6 NEWS2 (RCP, 2017b), Medium risk (NICE, 2007)</li></ul>

(Continued)

Table 1.2   (Continued)

Level of care	Criteria	Example
Level 2 Critical Care	• Patients needing pre-operative optimisation • Patients needing extended post-operative care • Patients stepping down to Level 2 from Level 3 • Patients receiving single organ support/basic respiratory support/basic cardiovascular support • Patients receiving advanced cardiovascular/renal/neurological/dermatological support	Bintu requires an arterial line and CVP line to be inserted to monitor her haemodynamic status prior to surgery. Keith has had a planned aortic aneurysm repair and requires hourly cardiovascular and haemodynamic monitoring due to the risk of haemorrhage and cardiac complications. Sally has received advanced respiratory support via invasive mechanical ventilation for sepsis and has been slow to wean off the ventilator. She requires continued respiratory monitoring and is at risk of deterioration. David has multiple intravenous vasoactive and rhythm control drugs to support cardiac output and tissue perfusion. He developed cardiogenic shock following myocardial infarction.
Level 3 Critical Care	Patients receiving advanced respiratory support alone or patients receiving a minimum of two organs supported	Tina was seen by the critical care outreach team as her NEWS2 was >7. She requires invasive mechanical ventilation for her respiratory and neurological dysfunction.

Critical care outreach teams

Critical care outreach teams (CCOTs) offer intensive care skills to patients with, or at risk of, critical illness or receiving care in locations outside the intensive care unit. CCOTs were instituted following the publication of *Comprehensive Critical Care* (Department of Health, 2000) in response to evidence that ward care of acutely deteriorating patients was suboptimal and that ward staff needed more support in their management. Many, but not all, hospitals in the UK now have some form of CCOT. NICE (2007) identifies that the response strategy for patients identified as being at risk of clinical deterioration should be triggered by either the physiological track and trigger score or clinical concern. CCOTs have three roles:

1. To identify and institute treatment in patients who are deteriorating within the hospital but outside of the ICU.
2. To help prevent admission to ICU or ensure that admission to a critical care bed happens in a timely manner to ensure best outcome.

3. To enable discharges from ICU by supporting the continuing recovery of discharged patients on wards and facilitating ward staff education.

In their 2018 review of available research, NICE found that there was some evidence of these objectives being met and they would continue to recommend consideration of providing access to a CCOT service for people in hospital at risk of deterioration.

NICE (2018) reports there is still much inconsistency in the service offered in terms of:

- Composition of outreach teams (that is, nurse-led or doctor-led, part of the cardiac arrest team or a separate entity).
- The way the teams are accessed.
- Whether these teams operate as a 7-day, 24-hour service or lesser periods.

ACVPU

Assessment of disability involves evaluating the function of the central nervous system. A rapid assessment of the patient's level of consciousness should be performed and it is recommended that the ACVPU tool is used for this. ACVPU is an acronym based on the previous tool AVPU with the addition of 'C' representing confusion. New-onset confusion, disorientation, delirium or any acute reduction in the Glasgow Coma Scale (GCS) score has been recognised by the Royal College of Physicians (2017) in NEWS2 as a sign potentially indicating serious deterioration. Assessment of new-onset confusion has also become part of the quick sequential organ failure assessment (qSOFA) in sepsis.

Using the ACVPU tool, the patient's response to stimuli is assessed and recorded:

A – the patient is alert

C – the patient presents with new-onset confusion, disorientation, delirium or acute reduction in GCS

V – the patient responds to verbal stimulus

P – the patient responds to painful stimulus

U – the patient is unresponsive

ACVPU should be assessed using a systematic approach, applying a range of stimuli to determine the optimal response from the patient. For example, if a patient responds to a verbal stimulus it is not necessary to apply a painful stimulus. If the patient has a reduced conscious level or new onset of confusion, a more comprehensive assessment is required. See Chapter 9 for discussion of use of the GCS score. This response to timely identification of patient deterioration needs to be communicated in an effective manner using a tool such as SBAR.

SBAR

Effective, structured communication will lead to timely assessment and management of the acutely ill person. SBAR is one tool that can facilitate this process and aid patient safety, and is used within this text to demonstrate its application. SBAR has four steps (NHS Institute for Innovation and Improvement, 2018):

Situation

Background

Assessment

Recommendation

SBAR acts as a memory prompt using a brief acronym that has been suggested and can reduce some of the communication barriers caused by hierarchy, gender, ethnic background or personal style of communication. It uses a common language platform during situations that require escalation or during critical events.

The components of a SBAR handover are:

- **S**ituation
    - o   Identify yourself, the patient by name and the site/unit you are calling from.
    - o   Describe your concern and the specific situation about which you are calling.
- **B**ackground
    - o   Give the patient's reason for admission and date.
    - o   Explain relevant medical history including prior procedures, current medications, allergies, pertinent laboratory results and other relevant diagnostic results.
- **A**ssessment
    - o   Provide vital signs and share subjective concerns. You may offer a provisional diagnosis.
- **R**ecommendation
    - o   Be specific about what you need and the timeframe.

Documentation of this conversation and when it took place is vital. Use of a tool such as SBAR has been recommended as it prevents vital information being missed or misinterpreted particularly in busy, clinically complex environments (Blom et al., 2015). Its use is also advocated more widely to improve nursing handover and communication (Cornell et al., 2014).

Person-centred care

The importance of using a person-centred approach in the application of a systematic ABCDE assessment has been highlighted. Ensuring that the person receiving care is involved in decision making is a key principle of the NHS constitution and is at the heart of each NICE clinical guideline. Informed consent and assessment of mental capacity where it is appropriate should be central to the delivery of high quality, evidence-based competent and compassionate care. There is a danger when considering care of the acutely unwell person that the physiological factors have pre-eminence – this text will seek to balance this with consideration of a holistic approach that acknowledges the vital support of the person, their family and carers from a psychological, social, ethical and spiritual perspective.

Patient safety

Underpinning all patient care interactions is the principle of patient safety. Patient safety is the avoidance of unintended or unexpected harm to people during the provision of healthcare. Implementing the systematic approaches to assessment, recognition and treatment outlined in this chapter will aid in delivering a safe approach that minimises avoidable harm to the patient. The healthcare practitioner needs to be aware of human factors that relate to technical skill performance such as fatigue and emotional wellbeing, and the role of non-technical skills such as communication, teamwork, leadership and situational awareness as factors in delivering safe patient care. These areas are beyond the remit of this text to consider in detail; however, further information can be found within the NHS England website at https://www.england.nhs.uk/patient-safety/.

SUMMARY

This chapter has outlined the ABCDE approach to assessing the acutely ill adult and highlighted the key national drivers relating to acute care practice. These will be referred to and their use demonstrated throughout the text.

	Initial Assessment (Look, Listen, Feel)	Measure	Action	Rationale/consider

A
AIRWAY
	Look and listen for signs of airway obstruction:
	
	• Foreign body, blood, vomit
	• Paradoxical chest and abdominal movements ('see saw' respirations), use of accessory muscles of breathing
	• Central cyanosis – late sign
	• Noisy breathing
	  o Snoring (tongue partial obstruction of upper airway)
	  o Stridor (narrowing/partial obstruction to upper airway)
	
	• Cervical spine injury
			• Obtain expert help immediately
			• Open the airway (head tilt, chin lift or jaw thrust)
			• Suction airway – only as far as can be visualised
			• Insertion of an oro/nasopharyngeal airway
			• Anticipate need for tracheal intubation
			• Commence high-concentration oxygen via non rebreathe mask 15l/min
				• Untreated, airway obstruction leads to lowered oxygen levels in the arterial circulation (hypoxaemia) and risk of hypoxic injury to the brain, kidneys, heart, cardiac and death (Resuscitation Council UK, 2021)

B BREATHING	Look, listen and feel for signs of respiratory distress: • Cyanosis • Accessory muscle usage • Assess depth, pattern, equal chest expansion • Listen to breath sounds • Percuss the chest • Auscultate the chest • Look for a raised jugular venous pressure (JVP) • Check the position of the trachea • Feel the chest wall to detect surgical emphysema (trapped air in tissues)	• Count the respiratory rate (normal rate is 12–20 breaths min) • Record the inspired oxygen concentration (%) • SpO_2	• Give oxygen, aim for target SpO_2 94–98%. For patients at risk of retaining carbon dioxide, aim for SpO_2 88–92%	• A high respiratory rate (25/min) is a marker of illness and a warning the patient may deteriorate suddenly • Consider ABG • Rattling airway noises indicate secretions caused by inability to cough sufficiently/take a deep breath • Wheeze/stridor suggest partial airway obstruction • Hyper resonance may suggest pneumothorax; dullness indicates consolidation or pleural fluid • Bronchial breathing indicates lung consolidation. Absent or reduced sounds indicate pneumothorax, pleural fluid or lung consolidation • A raised JVP indicates difficulty of blood returning to the heart via the superior vena cava • Tracheal deviation may indicate pneumothorax • Consider chest x-ray

(Continued)

	Initial Assessment (Look, Listen, Feel)	Measure	Action	Rationale/consider
C CIRCULATION	Look at the colour of the hands and digits: • Are they blue, purple, pink, pale or mottled? Assess the limb temperature • Are they cool or warm? Look for evidence of external or concealed haemorrhage Look for signs of fluid loss – vomiting, diarrhoea, bleeding, burns, drains	• Capillary Refill Time (CRT) (normal CRT is <2 seconds) • Palpate peripheral and central pulses for presence, rate, quality, regularity and equality (NEWS2 51–90bpm scores 0) • Blood pressure (BP) (NEWS2 systolic 111–219 mmHg scores 0) • Listen to heart sounds – does it correspond to pulse? Is there a murmur or pericardial rub (valve closure problem or heart surfaces rubbing together)? • Measure temperature (NEWS2 36.1–38°C scores 0) • Measure urine output (should be ≥0.5 ml/kg/min)	• Stop bleeding • Establish IV access • Take blood for routine haematological, biochemical, coagulation and microbiological investigations and cross matching • Give 500 ml bolus warmed crystalloid over less than 15 minutes if hypotensive. Use 250 ml for those with known cardiac failure • Reassess every 5 minutes, aiming for patient's normal BP or >100 mmHg • In primary chest pain and suspected Acute Coronary Syndrome (ACS) record 12-lead ECG early	• Normal skin is pink or brown with pink mucosa. Pale, blue or purple lips and mucosa indicates central cyanosis. Cool, blue tinged limbs indicates peripheral cyanosis • A prolonged CRT indicates poor peripheral perfusion • A weak, thready pulse indicates poor cardiac output • A bounding pulse may indicate sepsis • An irregular pulse indicates a possible cardiac arrhythmia, increased risk of embolus and/or impaired cardiac output • Consider 12 lead ECG • Blood pressure can be a late sign to change due to compensatory mechanisms, increased peripheral resistance in response to reduced cardiac output • Temperature >38°C or <36°C should raise suspicion of sepsis • Consider urinary catheter
D DISABILITY	Review and treat the ABCs: exclude or treat hypoxia and hypotension	• Examine the pupils (size, quality and reaction to light) • Assess conscious level using ACVPU (NEWS2 score 0 for A, 3 for CVPU) (see later discussion) or Glasgow Coma Scale • Measure blood glucose • Assess pain score using 0–3	• Check for reversible drug-induced causes of reduced consciousness. Give an antagonist where appropriate • Nurse unconscious patients in the lateral position until airway protected • Follow local protocol for hypoglycaemia management	• NOTE: Any patient with a decreased level of consciousness has a compromised airway • Hypoglycaemia can decrease conscious level
E EXPOSURE	To examine the patient properly, full exposure of the body may be necessary. Respect dignity and privacy, and minimise heat loss • Listen to the patient's story – relatives, friends, staff • Consider causes of any injury/trauma • Review patient notes and charts including prescribed items • Review blood results or radiological investigations Consider the level of care required by the patient (see discussion below)	• Examine the patient for signs of injury/trauma (bruising, bleeding, foreign objects in the body, abnormal or restricted movement, pain) • Examine pressure areas for evidence of pressure ulcer/development • Assess for peripheral or sacral oedema	• Treat and stabilise any injury • Record assessment findings, treatment and response	• Minimise any blood or fluid loss • Use the SSKIN bundle • Oedema is common in patients with heart failure

Figure 1.3 Overview of an ACBDE assessment

REFERENCES

Ali, M. (2018) Communication skills 5: Effective listening and observation. *Nursing Times*, 114 (4), 56–57.

Blom, L., Petersson, P., Hagell, P. & Westergren, A. (2015) The Situation, Background, Assessment and Recommendation (SBAR) model for communication between health care professionals: A clinical intervention pilot study. *International Journal of Caring Sciences*, 8 (3), 530–535.

Cornell, P., Townsend Gervis, M., Yates, L. & Vardaman, J. (2014) Impact of SBAR on nurse shift reports and staff rounding. *MedSurg Nursing*, 23 (5), 334–342.

Department of Health (2000) *Comprehensive Critical Care: A Review of Adult Critical Care Services*. London: Department of Health.

Intensive Care Society (ICS) (2021) *Levels of Adult Critical Care*. Second Edition. Available at: https://www.ics.ac.uk/Society/Patients_and_Relatives/Levels_of_Care (accessed 12 February 2022).

McQuillan, P., Pilkington, S., Allan, A., Taylor, B., Short, A., Morgan, G., Nielsen, M., Barrett, D. & Smith, G. (1998) Confidential inquiry into quality of care before admission to intensive care. *British Medical Journal*, 316, 1853–1857.

NHS Improvement (2016) *The adult patient who is deteriorating: Sharing learning from literature, incident reports and root cause analysis investigations*. Available at: https://improvement.nhs.uk/documents/176/Deterioration_in_adults_report_7july.pdf (accessed 26 June 2019).

NHS Institute for Innovation and Improvement (2018) *SBAR communication tool – Situation, Background, Assessment, Recommendation*. Available at: https://improvement.nhs.uk/resources/sbar-communication-tool/ (accessed 2 December 2019).

NICE (2007) *Acutely ill adults in hospital: Recognising and responding to deterioration*. Available at: www.nice.org.uk/guidance/cg50 (accessed 20 January 2022).

NICE (2014) *Safe staffing for nursing in adult inpatient wards in acute hospitals*. Available at: www.nice.org.uk/guidance/sg1 (accessed 20 January 2022).

NICE (2018) *Chapter 27. Critical care outreach teams. Emergency and acute medical care in over 16s: service delivery and organisation*. Available at: www.nice.org.uk/guidance/ng94/evidence/27.critical-care-outreach-teams-pdf-172397464640 (accessed 20 January 2022).

NICE (2019) *Hypertension in adults: Diagnosis and management*. Available at: www.nice.org.uk/guidance/ng136 (accessed 20 January 2022).

NMC (2018) *Future nurse: Standards of proficiency for registered nurses*. Available at: www.nmc.org.uk/globalassets/sitedocuments/education-standards/future-nurse-proficiencies.pdf (accessed 20 January 2022).

NPSA (2007) *Safer Care for the Acutely Ill Patient: Learning from Serious Incidents*. London: NPSA.

Resuscitation Council UK (2021) *The ABCDE approach*. Available at: https://www.resus.org.uk/library/abcde-approach (accessed 12 February 2022).

Royal College of Physicians (2017) *National Early Warning Score (NEWS) 2*. Available at: www.rcplondon.ac.uk/projects/outputs/national-early-warning-score-news-2 (accessed 26 June 2019).

2
UPPER AIRWAY – ANATOMY, PHYSIOLOGY AND PATHOPHYSIOLOGY

ALICE SKULL

Chapter learning outcomes

By the end of this chapter you will be able to:

1. Describe the location, structure and function of the nose, paranasal sinuses and pharynx.
2. Describe several protective mechanisms of the upper respiratory system.
3. Outline the causes of partial and complete airway obstruction.
4. Discuss the terms used to describe the respiratory sounds that indicate airway obstruction.

Key words

- Nose
- Nasal cavity
  - Olfactory mucosa
  - Respiratory mucosa
- Paranasal sinuses
- Pharynx
  - Nasopharynx
  - Oropharynx
  - Laryngopharynx

(Continued)

- Stridor
- Inspiratory and expiratory wheeze
- Gurgling
- Snoring
- Crowing

This chapter will consider the structure and function of the upper respiratory system in readiness for considering the management of airway obstruction in Chapter 3. The lower respiratory system is considered within Chapter 4 on breathing anatomy and physiology.

The respiratory system is divided into the upper and lower respiratory tract with its primary function to take up oxygen and expel carbon dioxide. The respiratory system includes the nose and paranasal sinuses, the pharynx, the larynx, the trachea, the bronchi and their smaller branches, and the lungs, which contain tiny air sacs called alveoli (Marieb & Hoehn, 2019). The upper respiratory system consists of all the structures from the nose to the larynx. The lower respiratory system consists of the larynx and all the structures below it (see Figure 2.1).

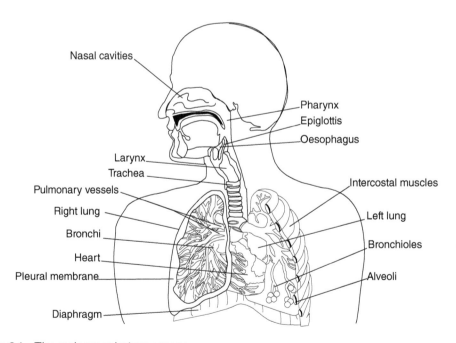

Figure 2.1   The major respiratory organs

Source: Reproduced with permission from Cook, N., Shepherd, A. & Boore, J. (2021) *Essentials of Anatomy and Physiology in Nursing Practice* (2nd ed.). London: SAGE.

Activity 2.1

Body organs are often described by their location and proximity to other body organs. Revise your understanding of the following terms before reading this chapter further:

- Anterior
- Inferior
- Superior
- Posterior

The nose:

- Provides an airway for respiration.
- Moistens and warms entering air.
- Filters and cleans inspired air.
- Serves as a resonating chamber for speech.
- Houses olfactory (smell) receptors.

During breathing, air enters the nasal cavity by passing through the nostrils. A small patch of olfactory mucosa lines the superior region of the nasal cavity and contains smell receptors. The respiratory mucosa lines most of the nasal cavity containing scattered goblet cells richly supplied with seromucous nasal glands. These glands contain cells that secrete a watery, sticky mucus containing an antibacterial enzyme (lysozyme) that traps inspired dust, bacteria and other debris, with the lysozyme destroying the bacteria. Natural antibiotics called defensins secreted from the mucosa help kill invading microbes. The high water content of the mucus film humidifies incoming air. Contaminated mucus is propelled gently towards the throat where it is swallowed and digested. When exposed to cold air this action becomes more sluggish and mucus accumulates in the nasal cavity leading to a runny nose on a cold winter's day. The nasal mucosa is richly supplied with sensory nerve endings, and contact with irritating particles such as dust and pollen triggers a sneeze reflex to expel irritants. Together with the nasal mucosa, the nasal conchae filter, heat and moisten the air and also act to reclaim heat and moisture during exhalation.

Five skull bones contain mucosa lined, air filled sinuses called 'paranasal sinuses', which lighten the skull and enhance the resonance of the voice, and may help moisten and warm the air (see Figure 2.2). The mucus they produce drains into the nasal cavity; the suction effect from blowing the nose aids in draining the sinuses.

The funnel shaped pharynx, about 13 cm in length, connects the nasal cavity and mouth superiorly to the larynx and oesophagus inferiorly. The pharynx is divided into three regions:

- Nasopharynx
- Oropharynx
- Laryngopharynx

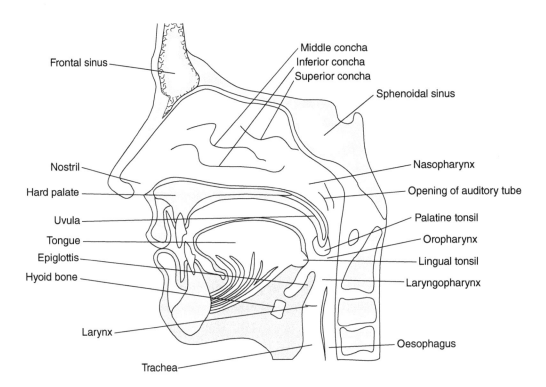

Figure 2.2   Regions of the pharynx

Source: Reproduced with permission from Cook, N., Shepherd, A. & Boore, J. (2021) *Essentials of Anatomy and Physiology in Nursing Practice* (2nd ed.). London: SAGE.

The nasopharynx lies above the point where food enters the body and serves only as an air passageway. During swallowing, the soft palate and uvula move superiorly to close off the nasopharynx and prevent food from entering the nasal cavity.

The oropharynx lies posterior to the oral cavity; both swallowed food and inhaled air pass through it. It has a more protective epithelium than the nasopharynx to accommodate the increased friction and chemical trauma of the passage of food.

The laryngopharynx also acts as a passageway for food and air and is similar in composition to the oropharynx. These areas also contain the tonsils, which are involved in protection against pathogens. When enlarged, the pharyngeal tonsils are referred to as adenoids.

Activity 2.2

Consider what effect infected and swollen adenoids have on the passage of air through the nasopharynx.

PATHOPHYSIOLOGY

Any obstruction or compromise to the airway can potentially be life threatening. Management and recognition of the patency of the airway is therefore the first parameter to be addressed in the ABCDE approach.

Obstruction of the airway may be partial or complete. It may occur at any level from the nose and mouth down to the trachea. In the unconscious patient, the commonest site of airway obstruction is at the level of the pharynx (Resuscitation Council UK, 2021). The pharynx may be occluded by the tongue, which falls backwards when the normal tone present in the muscles attaching the tongue to the jaw and floor of the mouth relaxes as a result of loss of consciousness. Obstruction may also be caused by vomit or blood, or as a result of regurgitation of gastric contents or trauma or foreign bodies.

Obstruction at laryngeal level may occur as a result of oedema of the structures of the upper airway as a result of burns, inflammation or anaphylaxis (see Chapter 7). Laryngeal spasm may be the result of an inappropriate response to upper airway stimulation, or due to an inhaled foreign body. The rapid nature of deterioration due to airway obstruction requires the healthcare practitioner to be proficient at detecting airway obstruction and the ability to respond appropriately.

Obstruction of the airway below the larynx is less common, but may arise from excessive bronchial secretions, mucosal oedema, bronchospasm, pulmonary oedema, aspiration of gastric contents or pulmonary haemorrhage and pneumothorax secondary to thoracic trauma (Resuscitation Council UK, 2021).

In partial airway obstruction, air entry is diminished and usually noisy. Inspiratory *stridor* (noise on breathing in) is caused by obstruction at the laryngeal level or above. Stridor is a high pitched wheezing sound caused by disrupted airflow. Sometimes it can almost seem to have a musical quality to it. Expiratory *wheeze*, however, suggests obstruction of the lower airways which tend to collapse and obstruct during expiration. A wheeze is a whistling sound, again often high pitched that is caused by a narrowed airway vibrating.

Other characteristic sounds that may be heard are:

- **Gurgling** – suggests presence of liquid or semisolid foreign material in the main airways.
- **Snoring** – arises when the pharynx is partially occluded by the tongue or the palate.
- **Crowing** – sound of laryngeal spasm (potentially life-threatening closure of the vocal chords). Called 'crowing' as the sound mimics the calling of crows.

Activity 2.3

Listen to a variety of respiratory sounds here: www.easyauscultation.com/course-contents?courseid=202.

Complete airway obstruction in a patient who is making respiratory effort results in paradoxical chest and abdominal movement, often described as '*see-saw breathing*'. Observation reveals that as the patient attempts to draw breath in, the chest lifts but the abdomen is drawn inwards. A normal breathing pattern would see synchronous movement upwards and outwards of the abdomen (pushed down by the diaphragm) and the rising of the chest wall. During airway obstruction other accessory muscles of respiration are also used, with the neck and shoulder muscles attempting to assist movement of the thoracic cage.

Remember!   Normal breathing should be quiet.

Obstructed breathing will be totally silent.

Noisy breathing indicates partial airway obstruction.

SUMMARY

The structure and function of the upper airway has been outlined. Recognition of obstruction of the airway is a key skill of the healthcare professional and requires swift action to address this life-threatening problem. The next chapter will consider how to manage obstruction of the airway.

There are further reading and resources available in preparation for the following chapters relating to management of the airway and breathing:

- Resuscitation Council UK provides guidance for healthcare professionals on the emergency management of airway obstruction and anaphylaxis: www.resus.org.uk/
- The Anaphylaxis Campaign provides in-depth information and helpline services: www.anaphylaxis.org.uk/

REFERENCES

Cook, N., Shepherd, A. & Boore, J. (2021) *Essentials of Anatomy and Physiology in Nursing Practice* (2nd ed.). London: SAGE.

Marieb, E. & Hoehn, K. (2019) *Human Anatomy and Physiology* (11th ed.). London: Pearson.

Resuscitation Council UK (2021) *The ABCDE approach*. Available at: https://www.resus.org.uk/library/abcde-approach (accessed 12 February 2022).

3

BREATHING – PATIENT-CENTRED APPROACHES TO AIRWAY MANAGEMENT: APPLICATION TO PRACTICE

SARAH MCGLOIN

Chapter learning outcomes

By the end of this chapter you will be able to:

1. Recognise a compromised airway.
2. Understand the manoeuvres to open an airway.
3. Know when to use a nasopharyngeal airway.
4. Know when to use an oropharyngeal airway.
5. Understand the use of a laryngeal mask.
6. Explain endotracheal intubation.
7. Discuss tracheostomy care.

Key words

- Airway
- Airway adjuncts
- Chin-lift head-tilt

INTRODUCTION

Whenever you are using the ABCDE approach to the deteriorating patient, the importance of 'A' for airway is constantly highlighted. A patent airway is one that is open and clear, where the patient is able to breath in oxygen and exhale carbon dioxide. A patient with a compromised airway may have received maxillofacial trauma, neck trauma or trauma directly to the trachea. Any compromised airway or airway obstruction is an emergency. Get expert help immediately. Untreated, airway obstruction results in hypoxia and risks damage to the major organs including the brain, kidneys and heart (Resuscitation Council UK, 2021). A blocked airway will result in cardiac arrest, and death. Unless the airway is patent and secured, no other interventions will be effective. This chapter will explain how to assess for and open a blocked or partially blocked airway. The chapter will then explain the use of the different airway adjuncts.

ASSESSING AN AIRWAY

To assess an airway, you need to adopt the following approach. Firstly, gently shake the individual by the shoulder and ask them loudly if they are okay. If they do not respond you need to assess for signs of airway obstruction using the 'look, listen, feel' approach (Resuscitation Council UK, 2021).

The oropharynx is the main location of upper airway obstruction. This is because if the tongue and jaw muscles are not functioning they cause the tongue and epiglottis to fall back. Also in an unconscious patient, there is less activity from the pharyngeal dilator muscles.

If the airway is obstructed, there will be see-saw respirations. This is also known as paradoxical chest and abdominal movement along with the use of the accessory respiratory muscles. When there is a complete obstruction of the airway there will be no breath sounds at the mouth or nose. The patient will be scared and look anxious and frightened. If there is a partial airway obstruction, there may be some air entry, but this is often noisy. If the patient is critically ill and has a GCS lower than 8, their airway will also be compromised. A late sign of airway obstruction is central cyanosis.

To assess the airway, the first thing to do is to kneel next to the patient and turn them onto their back. You then need to open up the airway. You can do this by a head tilt and chin lift. Place your hand on the patient's forehead and gently tilt the head back. Then place your fingertips under the patient's chin and lift the chin. The tongue can block the back of the throat when a person is unconscious. By doing the head tilt the anterior neck muscles are stretched and this lifts the tongue away from the posterior pharyngeal wall and draws the epiglottis forward as well. The tongue is pulled forward and the airway opens up. The chin lift stretches the muscles more and pulls the mandible and tongue forward. To summarise, this manoeuvre opens the airway by pulling the tongue forward. This is demonstrated in Figure 3.1.

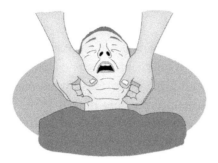 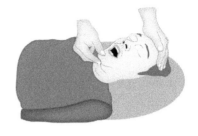

Figure 3.1 Jaw thrust and chin lift

If the patient's neck or spine has not been cleared and there is suspicion of a neck or spinal injury, it is advised to use the jaw thrust technique (Resuscitation Council UK, 2021). The aim of this manoeuvre is to move the jaw forward with minimal movement of the neck and spine.

This time, kneel at the head of the patient once they have been placed on their back. Position your fourth and fifth fingers underneath each side of the patient's jawbone (mandible). Keeping the head and neck stable, push each side of the patient's jawbone forward until the lower jaw is extended. Once the airway has been opened, you then need to look, listen and feel for any breaths. You can do this by kneeling next to the patient and placing your cheek near to their nose and throat whilst looking down at the patient, paying attention to their chest movements.

Look for chest wall movement and the presence of foreign objects. You can also look for evidence that the airway may become obstructed at a later time due to oedema such as singed facial or nasal hair, or sooty secretions that may indicate an inhalation injury.

Listen for breath sounds that may indicate an obstruction such as stridor, secretions and snoring.

Feel for a breath on the side of your cheek.

To secure an airway that may be at risk, it is important to understand which airway adjuncts to use when. The next section of this chapter will present a scenario for each of the airway adjuncts.

THE NASOPHARYNGEAL AIRWAY

The nasopharyngeal airway (NPA) is a simple airway adjunct. It is a soft rubber or plastic hollow, flexible tube with one end flared much like a trumpet and the other end that is bevelled. It is the bevelled end that is passed through the nose into the posterior pharynx. The larger the internal diameter of the airway, the longer the tube. A size 8.0–9.0 is used for a large adult, a 7.0–8.0 for a medium adult and a 6.0–7.0 for a small adult (Roberts et al., 2005).

It has advantages over the oropharyngeal airway (OPA) as it can be used in patients with an intact gag reflex, or oral trauma, that is, it can be used when it is difficult to use an oropharyngeal airway such as when a patient is intolerant of anything in their mouth or back of the throat. The nasopharyngeal airway is generally better tolerated than the oropharyngeal airway in a semi-conscious patient.

Consider the following case study:

Dominique Le Roux is a 25-year-old lady who had been involved in a high-speed road traffic accident where she had experienced some trauma, which required her to be sedated and ventilated. She has been on the critical care unit for the past 10 days, but is now semi-conscious with a GCS of 10 (E2 m5 v3).

- Dominique was able to say a few words.
- She has a very productive cough with purulent sputum upon suctioning. If she were not encouraged to cough, Dominique would simply lie in the bed and not cough. As a consequence the secretions were sitting at the back of her throat and pooling there with the risk of tracking down into her lower respiratory tract.

It was decided that Dominique would benefit from having a nasopharyngeal airway in place to help manage the secretions.

Sizing the nasopharyngeal airway

It is widely assumed that to size a NPA correctly, you compare the internal diameter of the tube with the patient's little finger or nostril size. The evidence base found this to be inaccurate. There is a relationship between NPA length and the height of the patient. Average height females require a size 6 NPA and males a size 7. Optimal and rapid sizing of the NPA can be modified from these average sizes to take account of the subject's height (Roberts et al., 2005).

It is important to get the size of the NPA correct. If it is too long, it may enter the larynx and irritate the cough reflex and cause the patient to cough and be intolerant of the tube, or it could even cause an airway obstruction. If it is too short, it will fail to separate the soft palate and tongue from the pharynx.

Inserting the nasopharyngeal airway

It is important to place the airway carefully so as not to cause intra-cranial placement. This needs to emphasise lifting the nostrils to reveal the nasal airway and the placement of the NPA parallel to the nasal floor, rather than in an upwards motion. It is important to lubricate and gently rotate the NPA, and try both nostrils. These will reduce any risk of the often quoted but very infrequent complication of intra-cranial tube placement (Roberts et al., 2005).

When inserting the airway into Dominique the following steps were undertaken:

- The airway and the need for the airway was explained to Dominique.
- Her oropharynx space was cleared of the oral secretions associated with her reduced level of consciousness.
- Dominique is a medium height lady and it was decided a size 6 airway would be suitable. As an additional check the size 6 tube was held against the side of her face. The tube extended from the tip of her nose to the tragus of the ear.
- Dominique's nostrils were lifted (as if she was 'sniffing the air') and opened to reveal her nasal passage. Having inspected both nostrils, it was decided to place the airway into her slightly larger nostril on the left.
- The NPA was lubricated with water-soluble lubricant to prevent soft tissue trauma on insertion.
- The NPA was inserted into the airway posteriorly parallel to the floor of the nasal cavity, and not with an upwards motion, with the bevel of the tip facing toward the nasal septum (i.e. with the pointed end lateral and the open end of the airway facing the septum). Gentle but firm pressure was used to pass the airway through the nasal cavity.
- There was a bit of resistance to the tube as it was being inserted. The NPA was then rotated slightly and re-advanced. There was still resistance and so the other nostril was tried and the tube was successfully passed.
- The airway was finally advanced straight back until the flange rested at the nostril opening.

Consider the following case study:

> Dominique had a significant collection of oral secretions that were sitting at the back of her throat. Due to her decreased level of consciousness, she was unable to cough effectively to clear the secretions. Dominique had:
>
> - Audible upper airway sounds.
> - Secretions you could feel if you placed your hands on her chest.
> - A moist rattling cough when stimulated.
>
> It was decided that Dominique would benefit from nasopharyngeal suctioning.

Nasopharyngeal suctioning

The nasopharyngeal tube provides easy access for the removal of secretions in the upper airway via suctioning.

Duration of use

There is no evidence for the ideal duration of NPA placement, however it is generally agreed that if it remains clinically indicated, an NPA can remain in place for up to 24 hours. However, to prevent pressure sores, it is good practice to alternate the NPA from one to the other nostril every six to eight hours. The nose should be inspected regularly for pressure areas around the flange of the NPA.

If the patient has copious pulmonary secretions requiring suction every hour or twice hourly, then inserting an NPA and leaving it in situ is warranted to permit easy access and to minimise trauma to the nasal mucosa from repeated insertion of the suction catheter.

Suctioning through an NPA

The procedure was explained to Dominique even though she was still only semi-conscious. It was important to explain what was about to happen, how long the procedure would be, what it would feel like and why it was necessary.

- The suction catheter was passed until Dominique produced a strong cough. The secretions were tapped.
- Care was taken not to go as far down as the carina.
- Suction was applied no longer than 15 seconds.
- If Dominique showed any signs of distress or there were large amounts of secretions suctioned, the catheter was partially withdrawn, giving Dominique a rest until she had recovered and was ready to continue.

THE OROPHARYNGEAL AIRWAY

Possibly better known than the NPA is the oropharyngeal airway (OPA). This is sometimes also referred to as the Guedel airway. The OPA is a curved hard plastic device that assists the maintenance of an airway in a patient with a decreased level of consciousness. As it is a hollow tube, it creates an opening from the mouth to the pharynx.

An OPA is used when there is a risk of airway obstruction as a result of relaxed muscles of the upper airway, or the airway being blocked by the tongue falling backwards into the space (Resuscitation Council UK, 2021). An OPA can help keep the tongue in place and also help when there is a need to manually ventilate a patient using a bag, valve and mask (BVM). The OPA can only be used in the unconscious patient as it can cause gagging and vomiting in those whose level of consciousness is increased.

Sizing the oropharyngeal airway

Although the OPA is easy to use, it is important that the correct size is used for the patient. If the OPA is too small, it will be occluded by the tongue and you will not be able to ventilate through it. If the OPA is too long, there is the risk of traumatic injury and laryngospasm. When choosing the size, the evidence suggests measuring the distance between the centre of the lips to the angle of the mandible.

Inserting the oropharyngeal airway

An OPA is only inserted into patients with a decreased level of consciousness (Resuscitation Council UK, 2021). If they are conscious, placing the device into their mouth could cause them to vomit or gag and possibly aspirate. It could also damage or dislodge teeth.

The OPA should be inserted into an adult using the rotation method:

1. Measure the OPA for the correct size.
2. Suction the oropharynx for possible obstructions.
3. Tilt the patient's head back and open the patient's mouth.
4. Hold the OPA at the flange with the tip pointing upwards towards the roof of the patient's mouth so that the device is actually upside down. This prevents it pushing the tongue back as the OPA is inserted.
5. Insert the OPA into the mouth above the tongue to approximately one-third of its length at the back of the throat.
6. Whilst continuing to gently insert the OPA, rotate it 180° until the curved part fits over the tongue and the tip points downwards, at the same time sliding it over the patient's tongue into the back of the pharynx until the flange touches the lips.
7. For a child, do not use the rotation method.

The OPA should slip gently into place. If there is resistance, stop and reposition the lower jaw and try again. Do not force the OPA into position as this can cause trauma to the mouth, teeth and upper airway.

Removing the oropharyngeal airway

An OPA should be removed immediately if the patient shows any signs of rejecting it through coughing, gagging or grabbing it (Resuscitation Council UK, 2021). The OPA is easily removed by sliding it out of the mouth following the natural curve of the mouth.

The OPA can be used to suction the upper airway. It can also keep the tongue in place and maintain an airway during BVM resuscitation.

THE LARYNGEAL MASK

The laryngeal mask airway (LMA) is an example of a supraglottic airway device (SAD). A SAD is positioned above or around the glottic opening but does not go any further down the airway. The purpose of a SAD is to maintain the upper airway clear from obstruction and is one of the most significant advances in airway management since the endotracheal (ET) tube. The LMA is used for patients with apnoea, severe respiratory failure, or impending respiratory arrest where endotracheal intubation is not possible (Mallett et al., 2013). It is also used for certain elective anaesthesia cases. LMAs can also be useful when a BVM ventilation is difficult when patients have severe facial deformity, a thick beard, or other factors that interfere with the face mask seal.

The LMA extends down the airway to just behind the epiglottis. Here the 'cuff' is inflated to create a seal behind the epiglottis, which both holds the airway open while also preventing fluids from entering either from above such as saliva or stomach contents entering from the oesophagus (Mallett et al., 2013). The volume of air required to inflate the cuff is unique for each brand, therefore the volume should always be checked before inflation.

The LMA is popular as it is less invasive than an endotracheal tube, decreases airway trauma, decreases neck mobility requirements, and has a reduced risk of laryngospasm and bronchospasm.

The first generation of LMA has since been replaced by second generations such as the i-gel. Unlike the inflatable LMA, the cuff of the i-gel is a soft elastomer, which conforms to fit the laryngeal structure of the casualty, creating a seal that way. Because there is no cuff, the insertion is significantly quicker. These second-generation devices include specific features to enhance positive pressure ventilation (PPV).

They also:

- Are designed to attempt to reduce the risk of aspiration by incorporating a channel for gastric decompression and suctioning secretions.
- Are more stable through a reinforced tip.
- Have a better seal under high pressure ventilation through improved cuff designs, which work better with higher ventilation pressures.
- Are more rigid in their design to prevent rotation and to facilitate easier insertion.

It is commonly thought that because the i-gel is thermoplastic, it expands to fit the casualty's airway in the same way that an inflatable LMA would. The material used in the i-gel is thermo-dynamic, which makes it soft and pliable, but it does not expand with heat.

Inserting the LMA

Firstly, select the appropriately sized LMA and note the maximum cuff inflation volume. Check the cuff for leaks.

- Completely deflate the cuff and apply a small amount of sterile, water-soluble lubricant to the posterior surface of the distal mask and cuff.
- Do a head-tilt chin lift to open the airway.
- Insert the tube into the mouth so that the mask opening is facing anteriorly. The standard approach is to manually guide the mask along the palates and into the throat by pushing with an index finger placed in the V-shaped notch where the tube attaches to the mask. Push the tube so that the lubricated posterior surface of the mask follows the curve of the palates. The mask should enter the hypopharynx along the posterior wall, to avoid deflecting and possibly causing a tube obstruction by the epiglottis. The mask is in the correct place when it sits over the laryngeal opening, and the tip of the mask will meet resistance to any further insertion.
- Release the hand from the tube before inflating the cuff.
- Inflate the cuff. Use half the recommended maximum cuff volume. As the mask sits over the glottic area, the tube will protrude 1 to 2 cm out of the mouth.
- Connect a bag-valve apparatus to the tube.
- Begin ventilation (8 to 10 breaths/minute, each about 500 mL and lasting about 1 second).
- Assess lung ventilation by auscultation and chest rise.
- Check end-tidal carbon dioxide to confirm placement.
- Fix the tube in place as appropriate.

Removing the LMA

Once the patient starts to complain about the presence of the LMA then it is time to take it out. This is done by deflating the cuff and simultaneously removing the LMA when the patient can open their mouth on command. Suction should be carried out prior to recovery of the reflexes or after removal of the LMA.

In the case of an i-gel, once consciousness is regained and the patient is coughing and swallowing, gently suction around the airway device. Once the patient is awake or easily rousable to voice, the i-gel can safely be removed by asking the patient to open their mouth wide and replacing it with an oxygen mask.

THE ENDOTRACHEAL TUBE

In certain circumstances, patients will require greater intervention to maintain a patent airway and also receive ventilatory support. In these instances, it will be necessary to insert an endotracheal tube through the mouth and into the trachea. This is the gold standard for securing an airway (Bersten & Handy, 2018). This will then be connected to a mechanical ventilator where the patient will receive invasive ventilation. The process of placing the tube within the trachea is called 'intubation'.

Endotracheal tubes come in a number of different sizes ranging from 2.0 millimetres (mm) to 10.5 mm in diameter. In general, a 7.0 to 7.5 mm diameter tube is often used for women and an 8.0 to 9.0 mm diameter tube for men. The tubes can either be single or double lumen.

Intubation and mechanical ventilation

A patient is intubated when they require respiratory support (Bersten & Handy, 2018). The rationale is to enable them to rest and to protect their airway whilst they receive interventions to support their organs and enhance their tissue perfusion. The endotracheal tube (ETT) helps maintain a patent airway and enables ventilation to take place.

The five main indications for intubation are:

1. Ventilatory support
2. Airway patency
3. Airway protection
4. Suctioning
5. Anaesthesia and surgery

Consider the following case study:

> Sadie Shah is a college student who has developed Type I respiratory failure as a result of a community-acquired pneumonia. Sadie has a very tight airway and an expiratory wheeze. She has a very productive purulent cough and is using her accessory muscles for respiratory support. Her ABGs are showing a significant respiratory acidosis. Sadie is developing hypoxaemia and becoming confused. She is looking physically tired. The decision has been made to intubate Sadie.

The intubation procedure

Once it was decided Sadie required intubation, the nurse's role in intubation was to work as a member of the interprofessional team, to assist in the procedure and to ensure the correct equipment was obtained and prepared whilst Sadie was being ventilated and oxygenated with BVM ventilation. Sadie was paced in the supine position with her head slightly hyperextended in a 'sniffing' position. The bed was positioned to enable the anaesthetist who was intubating Sadie to easily access Sadie's mouth. Once intubated, the tube was secured using a specific endotracheal tubes (ETT) holder and the length of the tube at Sadie's lips noted (Bersten & Handy, 2018). This should be assessed regularly to ensure the ETT had not slipped out of position. A chest X-ray was performed to ensure the tube was in the correct position located just above the carina.

Basic intubation equipment

Personal protective equipment (gloves, face shield or goggles)

Laryngoscope handle

Assortment of various sizes of laryngoscope blades

Spare batteries and bulbs for the laryngoscope

Various sizes of oropharyngeal airways

Yankauer suction

Stylet to provide more rigidity and/or allow for adjusting the curve of the ETT

Various sizes of ETT appropriate for the patient

10 ml syringe to inflate the cuff on cuffed ETT

ETT holder to secure the tube

Water-soluble lubricant to lubricate the cuff

Magill forceps to assist in nasotracheal intubation

Gum elastic bougie (intubating introducer or 'tube changer')

End tidal CO_2 monitor to determine proper placement of the ETT in the trachea

Stethoscope

Care of the endotracheal tube

One of the key interventions when caring for an intubated patient like Sadie is to monitor the cuff pressure to ensure there is an adequate seal between the cuff and the trachea, without causing pressure and necrosis to the tracheal mucosa. The cuff is the inflatable balloon towards the end of the tube. The cuff pressure needs to be recorded four hourly using a cuff manometer and needs to remain between 15 and 22 mmHg (Lorente et al., 2014).

Some patients benefit from what is known as a 'subglottic ETT'. This is helpful for patients who have secretions pooling above the cuff and which may track down to contribute to a ventilator-acquired pneumonia. This type of tube has a suction port that sits above the cuff and low level suction is applied to this to remove the secretions (Frost et al., 2013).

Sadie received sedation whilst she was intubated and ventilated. As a result, she was unable to blink and so required frequent eye care. Sadie also required frequent mouth care. The ETT also required humidification to prevent secretions building up on the plastic wall and occluding the lumen. Suctioning of secretions was also necessary. This will be discussed further in the section on tracheostomy care.

THE TRACHEOSTOMY TUBE

The final airway adjunct to consider is the tracheostomy tube.

Consider the following case study:

> Rohit Sharma is a 35 year old who had been on the critical care unit for a number of weeks with multi-organ dysfunction caused by sepsis. He has recently been transferred to the ward but has a tracheostomy tube in situ. Rohit's tracheostomy was inserted to make it more comfortable for him whilst he was being ventilated for a prolonged period of time.

Tracheostomies are beneficial as they have a decreased risk of laryngeal damage and there is reduced airway resistance and dead space, making breathing easier. They are more comfortable and less sedation is required. Communication is easier (Bersten & Handy, 2018).

There are a variety of tracheostomy tubes available. Fenestrated ones aid communication, while those with an inner cannula help with secretion build up.

Tracheostomy care

The nursing care of Rohit included caring for his tracheostomy. The stoma needed to remain free from infection and required cleaning with saline, and the absorbent foam dressing that sat under the flange and fixation device was changed at least 12 hourly. This is a two-person job.

Humidification

The tracheostomy tube needs to receive heated (to body temperature) humidification to prevent secretion build up and occlusion. Humidification aims to warm and moisten inspired air.

Humidifiers are either passive or active. A passive humidifier is known as a heat and moisture exchange filter (HME) (Bersten & Handy, 2018). Rohit had one of these in situ when he went for investigations such as a scan or was being mobilised by the physiotherapist. As Rohit exhaled, the warm moist air condensed within the membrane of the HME, trapping water.

When Rohit was at his bedspace, he was attached to an active humidifier that sat in inspiratory limb of the circuit. The gas flows through heated water, which humidifies the gas.

Suctioning

Rohit required regular tracheal suctioning. This is the removal of secretions using a negative pressure through a suction catheter. The aim is to aspirate and remove secretions. This prevented atelectasis and airway obstruction whilst enhancing gaseous exchange and oxygenation.

Rohit's tracheostomy tube was suctioned when indicated by signs such as:

- Visible or audible secretions
- Reduced chest movements
- Reduced air entry
- Course crackles
- Reduced oxygen saturations
- Coughing or increased work of breathing

There are different suctioning devices. Suctioning can take place as open suctioning where the suction catheter is passed directly into the tube, having disconnected the patient from the ventilator or oxygen. Closed suction on the other hand has the suction catheter attached to the tube and circuit and is fed through a plastic sleeve without the need to disconnect from the ventilator or oxygen supply. Suctioning should only take 15 seconds using a continuous suction technique at a suction pressure of less than 150 mmHg (Mallet et al., 2013). The potential complications associated with suctioning are listed as:

- Hypoxia/hypoxaemia
- Bronchoconstriction
- Bleeding
- Atelectasis
- Cardiovascular instability

Rohit's tracheostomy tube was finally removed once he was in the ward, had an effective cough and was less reliant on the support of the tracheostomy tube. The tube was removed following local Trust policy.

SUMMARY

This chapter has presented a variety of airway management techniques and adjuncts. A number of case studies have been used to apply airway management principles to practice. The following chapter will now proceed to explore 'B' for breathing.

REFERENCES

Bersten, A.D. & Handy, J. (2018) *Oh's Intensive Care Manual* (8th ed.). Oxford: Elsevier.

Frost, S.A., Azeem, A., Alexandrou, E., Tam, V., Murphy, J.K., Hunt, L., O'Regan, W. & Hillman, K.M. (2013) Subglottic secretion drainage for preventing ventilator associated pneumonia: A meta-analysis. *Australian Critical Care*, 26 (4), 180–188.

Lorente, L., Leucona, M., Jimenez, A., Lorenzo, L., Roca, I., Carera, J., Llanos, C. & Mora, M.L. (2014) Continuous endotracheal tube pressure control system protects against ventilator-acquired pneumonia. *Critical Care*, 18 (2), R77.

Mallett, J., Albaran, J. & Richardson, A. (2015) *Critical Care Manual of Clinical Procedures and Competencies*. Chichester: Wiley-Blackwell.

Resuscitation Council UK (2021) *2021 resuscitation guidelines*. Available at: www.resus.org.uk/library/2021-resuscitation-guidelines (accessed February 2022).

Roberts, K., Whalley, H. & Bleetman, A. (2005) The nasopharyngeal airway: Dispelling myths and establishing facts. *Emergency Medicine Journal*, 22, 394–396.

4

BREATHING – ANATOMY, PHYSIOLOGY AND PATHOPHYSIOLOGY

SARAH MCGLOIN

Chapter learning outcomes

By the end of this chapter you will be able to:

1. Label a diagram of the respiratory tract.
2. Identify the key components of the lower respiratory tract.
3. Describe the movement of gases into and out of the lungs.
4. Discuss the major lung volumes.
5. Describe how oxygen is used by the cells to produce energy.
6. Demonstrate a systematic approach to arterial blood gas analysis.
7. Differentiate between Type I and Type II respiratory failure.

Key words

- Respiration
- Ventilation
- Transport of gases
- Oxygen dissociation curve
- Cellular respiration
- Arterial blood gas

INTRODUCTION

The function of the respiratory system is primarily gas exchange. We need to breathe not only to take in oxygen, but to excrete carbon dioxide via the lungs. The respiratory system also has a metabolic function in that it also removes carbon dioxide, a waste by-product of energy production in the cells. Constant levels of carbon dioxide within the blood and the tissues are necessary to maintain the driving force that keeps us breathing and taking on oxygen. However, too much carbon dioxide in the blood will impact on the production of energy, to the point where life could be threatened. This chapter will explore the anatomy and physiology of the respiratory system along with underlying pathophysiology related to respiratory failure. The chapter will conclude with a systematic approach to arterial blood gas analysis.

RESPIRATORY ANATOMY

An overview of the respiratory system can be seen in Figure 4.1. The upper respiratory tract commences at the nasal cavity. This is a large cavity lined with cilia and glandular epithelium, which

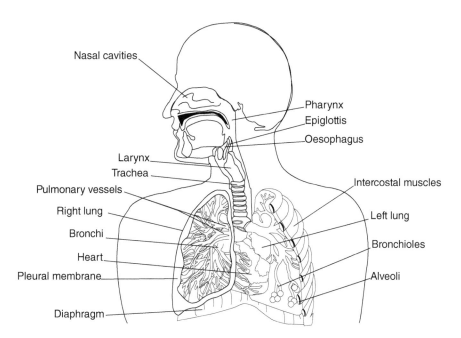

Figure 4.1 The respiratory tract

Source: Reproduced with permission from Cook, N., Shepherd, A. & Boore, J. (2021) *Essentials of Anatomy and Physiology in Nursing Practice* (2nd ed.). London: SAGE.

filters, heats and moistens air on inspiration (Peate, 2018). The cavity's surface area is increased by a number of projections called 'conchae'. The conchae continue throughout the throat cavities and the pharynx, which has two components – the oropharynx and the nasopharynx. The Nasopharynx is an extension of the throat upwards towards the nasal passages. The oropharynx opens into the oesophagus and the glottis, which is an opening to the lungs. The epiglottis prevents food entering the glottis when swallowing (Tortora & Derrickson, 2017).

Having passed through the glottis, air moves into the larynx (McLafferty et al., 2013a). This structure is supported by muscles that suspend the larynx from a bone in the neck called the 'hyoid'. The larynx consists of folds of cartilage, which form the vocal cords. From the larynx, the air moves into the trachea. This is around 12 cms long and 2.5 cms wide (Peate, 2018). This tube of fibrous and muscular tissue is strengthened by 16–20 C-shaped cartilage rings, which prevent it from collapsing (Peate, 2018). There is no cartilage at the back as this prevents friction with the oesophagus during swallowing. Again, the trachea is lined with cilia and mucus-producing epithelium. The mucus helps moisten the airways but also traps dust particles and micro-organisms that may have been inhaled. These particles are wafted in mucus by the cilia towards the glottis, where the mucus is swallowed and the particles destroyed (McLafferty et al., 2013a).

The trachea divides into smaller and smaller airways (Tortora & Derrickson, 2017). These form the lower respiratory tract, the structures of which can be seen in Figures 4.2 and 4.3.

- The left and right primary bronchi. These are similar to the trachea, but of a smaller diameter.
- Secondary bronchi branch from the primary bronchi and each supplies a lobe of the lungs.
- The secondary bronchi branch to form the tertiary bronchi, which are smaller bronchi.
- The tertiary bronchi branch into bronchioles. These are less than 1 mm in diameter and divide further to form an extensive network of bronchioles. These are made up of smooth muscle with no cartilage.
- The bronchioles terminate in alveolar ducts. These open into minute clusters of globular sacs called 'alveoli'. There are approximately 300 million alveoli in total. Each alveolus is 0.3 mm in diameter and made up of elastic tissue. The alveoli have an extensive blood supply. This respiratory membrane formed by the capillary endothelial cells and the alveoli epithelium provides the site of gas exchange between the lungs and the circulation (McLafferty et al., 2013a).

The lungs are paired organs located within the thoracic cavity. The left lung has two lobes to make room for the heart within the thoracic cavity, whilst the right lung has three. The lungs and the chest wall are lined with the visceral and parietal membranes. The thin cavity between these membranes forms the pleural space, which is filled with pleural fluid. The lungs are separated from the abdomen by the diaphragm. This is the main respiratory muscle that is dome-shaped just before lung expansion and flattens during breathing, which is essential for lung inflation and deflation, and are driven by the phrenic nerve. The other key respiratory muscles are the intercostal muscles, which are driven by the intercostal nerves (Peate, 2018).

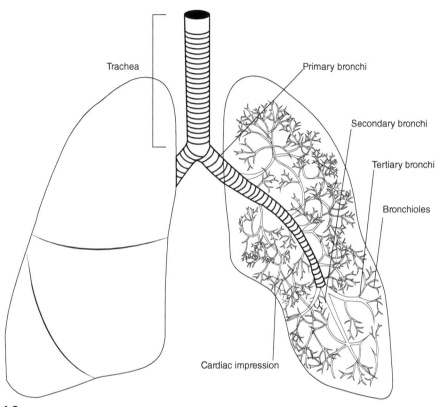

Figure 4.2

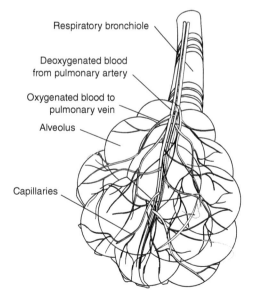

Figure 4.3

RESPIRATORY PHYSIOLOGY

Air contains several gases and each gas exerts its own pressure, which is known as a partial pressure. Collectively, the gases make up the total pressure of the mixture of gases. Clinically, the partial pressure of respiratory gases is expressed in kilopascal (kPa). To understand the movement of gases at the lungs, it is helpful to consider the three gas laws that relate to how gases act in a mixture and under pressure (Tortora & Derrickson, 2017):

1. **Boyles Law** (inspiration)
   The pressure exerted by a gas is inversely proportional to the size of a container.
2. **Dalton's Law** (alveolar air)
   The pressure exerted by a mixture of gases is the sum total of the partial pressures and the pressure exerted by each gas is proportional to its percentage representation.
3. **Henry's Law** (diffusion at the membrane)
   The concentration of a gas dissolved in a liquid is proportional to its partial pressure. The solubility of a gas will also depend on its solubility coefficient. Carbon dioxide is 20 times more soluble than oxygen.

THE MOVEMENT OF GASES

The movement of gases into and out of the body is achieved by four processes:

1. Pulmonary ventilation.
2. Gas exchange across the respiratory membrane – external respiration.
3. Transport of gases to the tissues and cells.
4. Gas exchange at the tissues – internal respiration (McLafferty et al., 2013a).

Pulmonary ventilation

Pulmonary ventilation involves inspiration and expiration and the movement of air from the atmosphere into the alveoli. Inspiration is an active process where the size of the thoracic cavity is increased. Contraction of the diaphragm flattens the base of the cavity. As the intercostal muscles contract, they lift the rib cage up and out. This causes the size within the thoracic cavity to increase and the pressure in the lungs to fall below atmospheric pressure. This forms a pressure gradient between the atmosphere (760 mmHg) and the lungs (758 mmHg). Air is drawn into the thoracic cavity down the gradient. This relates to Boyles law, which states that the pressure exerted by a gas is inversely proportional to the size of a container (Tortora & Derrickson, 2017).

As inspiration starts, the gas moves through the airway to the lungs. These are divided into the conducting zone and the respiratory zone. The conducting zone including the nasal cavity, pharynx, trachea, bronchi and bronchioles form the anatomical dead space, which means they do not take part in gas exchange – 150 mls of gas sits in this space (Tortora & Derrickson, 2017). External respiration takes place in the respiratory zone and is the exchange of gases at the alveoli. Some alveoli may not be available for this due to poor perfusion or atelectasis. These become the physiological dead space. Lung disease increases the physiological dead space and impairs gas exchange (McLafferty et al., 2013a). The lungs do not fully deflate on expiration with the alveoli and airways being filled with gas left over from the last breath. This prevents the airways from collapsing and is known as the functional residual volume (which is approximately 2400 mls). The tidal volume is the volume of each breath and is approximately 500 mls (8–10 mls/kg) (Tortora & Derrickson, 2017).

In normal ventilation, expiration is passive and occurs due to the recoil of the respiratory muscles. The size of the thoracic cavity decreases so the pressure of the gas in the lungs is greater than that of atmospheric pressure. The pressure gradient is reversed and air rushes out of the thoracic cavity. As well as the diaphragm, the muscles of the neck and the abdomen play an important role in inspiration and expiration. Expiration may become a forced active process during laboured breathing (Tortora & Derrickson, 2017).

The diaphragm is responsible for 80% of the muscular activity associated with breathing at rest and commands only 3% of the total body energy expenditure. During exercise this can increase to 30% or more (Tortora & Derrickson, 2017). Severe lung disease can require so much energy that the individual is unable to mobilise. As with any muscle, the diaphragm can get tired, resulting in an accumulation of lactic acid. This is seen in severe asthma (McLafferty et al., 2013a).

Chemical control of ventilation

Breathing is controlled by the respiratory centre in the pons and medulla of the central nervous system (Peate, 2018). Carbon dioxide (CO_2) is the main stimulus for breathing. Chemoreceptors in the medulla, carotid sinus and aortic arch inform the respiratory centre when the CO_2 levels require adjustment (McLafferty et al., 2013b). The medulla also reacts to changes in pH levels within the cerebral spinal fluid. A drop in oxygen (O_2) also stimulates the chemoreceptors (McLafferty et al., 2013b). This is summarised in Table 4.1.

Table 4.1   Control of breathing

Stimulus	CNS activity	Physiological response
High CO_2	Stimulates the respiratory centre	Increased rate and depth of breathing
Low CO_2	Depresses the respiratory centre	Shallow breathing or even apnoea, until the CO_2 accumulates
High body temperature	Stimulates the respiratory centre	Increases respiratory rate
Low body temperature	Depresses the respiratory centre	Decreases respiratory rate

Pressure relationships in the thoracic cavity

The lungs contain elastic fibres and have a natural tendency to recoil and collapse. A small negative pressure within the pleural space prevents this. This negative pressure is always present throughout the respiratory cycle. It is generated from:

1.   The parietal pleura being attached to the chest wall and being pulled outwards.
2.   The visceral pleura being attached to the lung surface and pulling inwards as the lung tries to recoil.
3.   A small amount of pleural fluid is present between the two layers. This helps the pleura move smoothly over each other and creates adhesive forces between the two. The drainage of this fluid by the lymphatic system creates a suction and maintains this negative pressure within the pleural space.

The role of surfactant

Gas reaching the alveoli contains water. If water were placed on the alveoli's surface, surface tension forces would develop and the alveoli would collapse. To prevent water lining the lung and forming surface tension that would cause the alveoli to collapse, Type II cells within the lungs produce surfactant (Credland, 2017).

Surfactant is a lipoprotein, with a hydrophobic portion and a hydrophilic portion. The alveoli are lined with the hydrophobic portion outermost so that water is repelled from the surface of the alveoli. This lowers the surface tension of the alveoli and prevents it from collapsing (Clancy & McVicar, 2009).

Surfactant is also to control the size of the alveoli. The larger the alveoli, the thinner the layer of surfactant and the greater the surface tension that will cause the alveoli to collapse inwards. The smaller the alveoli, the thicker the surfactant and the lower the surface tension expands the alveoli (Clancy & McVicar, 2009).

The work of breathing

Lungs have to overcome opposing forces to be able to inflate. This is known as the 'work of breathing'. These forces are:

1. Airway resistance, this is the resistance that air encounters as it is drawn into the airways.
2. Elastic recoil.
3. Surface tension.
4. Viscera of the lung.
5. Weight of the thoracic cavity.

Pulmonary capacities and volumes

Understanding capacities and lung volumes can help in the diagnosis of altered physiology within the lungs. There are a number of pulmonary capacities and volumes (Tortora & Derrickson, 2017), which are presented in Figure 4.4.

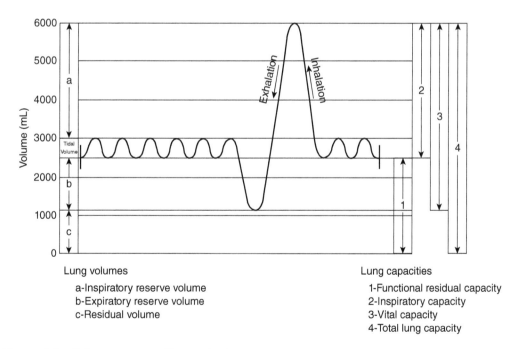

Figure 4.4   Pulmonary capacities and volumes

Vital capacity is the maximum amount that is breathed out after filling the lungs first and is around 4600 mls.

Inspiratory capacity relates to a deep inspiration and is the vital capacity plus the inspiratory reserve volume, and is around 3500 mls.

Functional residual capacity is the amount of air that remains in the lungs at the end of a normal breath and is 2300 mls. Total lung capacity is the greatest volume that the lungs can be expanded with the greatest respiratory effort and is around 5800 mls.

Tidal volume is the normal depth of breath in or out and is 8–20 mls/kg.

Inspiratory reserve volume is a normal breath in and then breath in again. It is the extra volume of air that can be inspired over and above the normal tidal volume so about 3000 mls.

Expiratory reserve volume is a breath out and then out again. The extra volume that can be breathed out after a normal tidal volume is around 1100 mls.

Residual volume is the volume of gas left in the lungs after forced expiration, which is around 1200 mls (Tortora & Derrickson, 2017).

External respiration

External respiration is the movement of oxygen from the alveoli into the circulation and the movement of carbon dioxide from the blood into the alveoli, and is dependent on gas exchange and ventilation in the respiratory zone. This must match carbon dioxide production. Increasing the dead space will decrease alveolar ventilation and may result in hypercapnia. Therefore, the rate of alveolar ventilation controls levels of alveolar carbon dioxide and in turn the partial pressure of carbon dioxide exerted within the blood ($PaCO_2$). The blood in the alveolar capillaries is also oxygenated during external respiration. The movement of gases is dependent on gas concentration (McLafferty et al., 2013b).

Both oxygen and carbon dioxide move by diffusion down a concentration gradient, from an area of high concentration to an area of low concentration. This is how carbon dioxide is removed from the blood as oxygen enters the blood.

The partial pressure of carbon dioxide in the alveoli is 5.3 kPa, whilst it is 6.1 kPa in the capillaries at the alveoli. This concentration difference allows carbon dioxide to diffuse from the capillaries across the alveolar membrane into the alveoli. The oxygen concentration in inspired air is 13.3 kPa which is higher than that in the capillary, which is 5.3 kPa. This concentration gradient allows the oxygen to diffuse across the alveolar membrane into the capillaries at the lungs (McLafferty et al., 2013b).

Small tidal volumes will encourage lung collapse and lead to hypoxia. Increasing the $PaCO_2$ can be achieved through keeping the lungs open for more time or increasing the $PaCO_2$ (Henry's Law).

However poor solubility of oxygen and the nature of the oxygen dissociation curve means that increasing the PaO_2 once saturation exceeds 90–93% will have little effect on the total PaO_2 (McLafferty et al., 2013b).

Transport of gases

Oxygen

About 1 litre of oxygen is transported to the cells every minute. 1.5% of oxygen is dissolved in the plasma but 98.5% is attached to the haemoglobin in red blood cells. This forms oxyhaemo-globin. Haemoglobin is an oxygen-carrying protein. Haem contains the iron molecule, which gives red blood cells their colour. Globin is a protein to which haem is attracted. In the pulmonary capillaries where the partial pressure of oxygen is high, haemoglobin binds readily with the oxygen until all the binding sites are saturated. In the tissue capillaries, the partial pressure of oxygen is lower and less oxygen bids to the haemoglobin thus freeing it up to diffuse from the capillaries into the cells (Tortora & Derrickson, 2017).

The increasing level of carbon dioxide in the tissues encourages the release of oxygen from the haemoglobin. This is important in exercise where the carbon dioxide levels in muscle tissues rises therefore encouraging oxygen to be released at the tissues.

The oxygen dissociation curve

Several factors influence the binding of oxygen with the haemoglobin and this is represented by the oxygen dissociation curve presented in Figure 4.5, which shows the extent of saturation of haemoglobin for a given pressure of oxygen. Increasing the pressure of oxygen increases the saturation of haemoglobin with oxygen. The line is curved. The plateau of the curve demonstrates that once the haemoglobin is saturated above 90% with oxygen, a higher partial pressure of oxygen is needed to increase the saturation of oxygen. On the steep portion of the curve, it is seen that small changes in the partial pressure of oxygen (or oxygen concentration) causes large changes in haemoglobin saturation with oxygen. When the curve shifts to the right, haemoglobin will give up oxygen more easily. This is known as the Bohr effect (Tortora & Derrickson, 2017).

Blood pH affects the affinity of oxygen to haemoglobin. Low pH increases the affinity whilst alkalinity decreases it. As has been discussed, higher than normal levels of carbon dioxide increase the blood acidity and decrease the oxygen's affinity to haemoglobin. An increased temperature decreases the affinity of oxygen to haemoglobin, whilst a reduced temperature increases the affinity (Tortora & Derrickson, 2017).

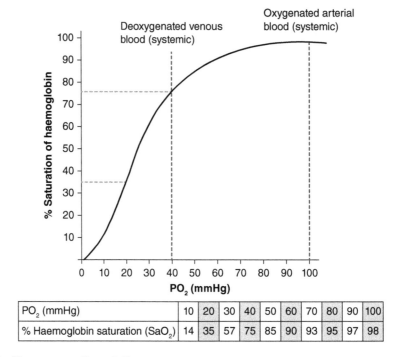

PO$_2$ (mmHg)	10	20	30	40	50	60	70	80	90	100
% Haemoglobin saturation (SaO$_2$)	14	35	57	75	85	90	93	95	97	98

Figure 4.5   The oxygen dissociation curve

Carbon dioxide

Carbon dioxide is a waste product of internal respiration. Blood arriving at the arterial end of the capillary is low in carbon dioxide and therefore carbon dioxide diffuses out of the cell into the capillary. Carbon dioxide is transported in three ways:

1. Dissolved in plasma (7%)
2. Attached to haemoglobin (23%)
3. As bicarbonate (70%)

Carbon dioxide (23%) is mainly transported on the protein part of haemoglobin rather than the haem portion, 7% is dissolved in plasma. Most however is transported on bicarbonate. This requires a chemical reaction, which takes place in the red blood cells. The carbon dioxide diffuses into the red blood cells where it combines with water to form carbonic acid. This then splits to form bicarbonate and hydrogen ions. Some of the bicarbonate diffuses back into the plasma (Tortora & Derrickson, 2017). This is shown in Figure 4.6.

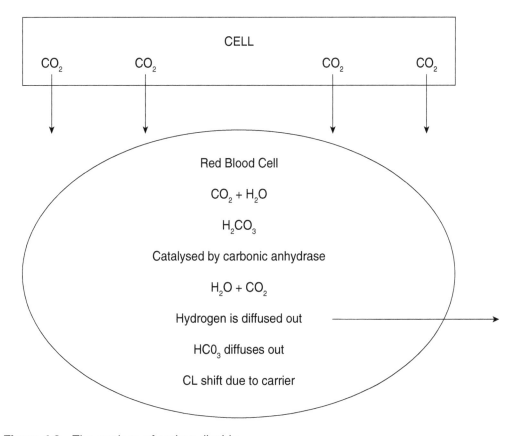

Figure 4.6   The carriage of carbon dioxide

When blood reaches the lungs, the chemical reaction that resulted in the formation of bicarbonate and hydrogen is reversed and they recombine to form carbonic acid, which then splits to form carbon dioxide and water. Carbon dioxide then diffuses out of the red blood cell into the plasma where it can then diffuse across the capillary membrane into the alveoli to be excreted (Tortora & Derrickson, 2017).

Internal respiration

Once external respiration has taken place at the lungs and the oxygen and carbon dioxide transported to the tissues, internal respiration occurs. This is the movement of oxygen from the blood in the capillaries into the cells of the tissues and the movement of carbon dioxide – the waste product of cellular respiration – from the tissue cells into the blood at the capillaries (McLafferty et al., 2013b). This again occurs due to a concentration gradient.

The oxygenated blood entering the capillaries at the tissues has a partial pressure of 13.3 kPa whilst the partial pressure of oxygen in the cells is 5.3 kPa (McLafferty et al., 2013b). Oxygen therefore diffuses from the blood in the capillary through the capillary membrane into the cells until equilibrium is achieved. In contrast, carbon dioxide levels in the blood entering the tissues is 5.3 kPa whilst in the cells is higher at 6.1 kPa. Carbon dioxide therefore diffuses from the cells into the blood in the capillaries until equilibrium is achieved (McLafferty et al., 2013b). At the end of internal respiration, blood is deoxygenated and the partial pressure of oxygen is 5.3 kPa and 6.1 kPa for carbon dioxide. This deoxygenated blood then returns to the lungs via the venous system where external respiration once again takes place (McLafferty et al., 2013b).

Cellular respiration

Cellular respiration takes place within the cytoplasm and the mitochondria of the cells. Aerobic respiration involves oxygen being used to produce energy in the form of adenosine triphosphate (ATP). The chemical equation for cellular respiration is:

$$C_6H_{12}O_6 \; 6O_2 + 6CO_2 + 6H_2O + 38 \; ATP$$

There are three stages to cellular respiration:

1. Glycolysis
2. The citric acid cycle
3. Electron transport/oxidative phosphorylation

Stage 1 Glycolysis

This takes place in the cytoplasm of the cell. Here, glucose, which is a six-carbon molecule, splits into two three-carbon molecules to form 'pyruvate'. During glycolysis, two molecules of ATP and two high energy carrying molecules called 'nicotinamide adenine dinucleotide hydrogen' (NADH) (Tortora & Derrickson, 2017) are formed.

Stage 2 The citric acid cycle

This takes place in the matrix of the mitochondria. The pyruvate from glycolysis moves into the matrix of the mitochondria. This is then split into two and releases carbon dioxide whilst forming the molecule acetyl. The acetyl then attaches to a co-enzyme A to form acetyl co-A, 2 NADH and CO_2. The acetyl co-A combines with a four-carbon molecule called 'oxaloacetic acid' to form a six-carbon molecule. Throughout the citric acid cycle, the six-carbon molecule is broken back down into the four oxaloacetic acid. ATP, NADH and FADH2 are all produced as this process takes place, as is carbon dioxide (Tortora & Derrickson, 2017).

Stage 3 Electron transfer chain/oxidative phosphorylation

This takes place in the membrane of the cristae of the mitochondria. Here NADH and FADH2 release electrons to become NAD and FAD. These electrons move down an electron transfer chain, releasing energy. This energy is used to pump proton electrons out of the matrix of the mitochondria. This causes a concentration gradient with more protons outside the membrane than inside it. Therefore, the hydrogen moves back across the membrane through diffusion. At the same time, this synthesises ATP. At the end of this electron transfer chain, oxygen accepts hydrogen to form water (Tortora & Derrickson, 2017).

Arterial blood gas analysis

Arterial blood gas (ABG) analysis can be used to assess respiratory function, gas exchange and acid base status as well as to provide immediate information about electrolytes (Woodrow, 2004). It is a diagnostic adjunct that can indicate tissue perfusion but should not blinker clinical judgement. An ABG measures the partial pressure of oxygen and carbon dioxide as well as the pH, bicarbonate level and base excess levels (Coleman & Morozowich, 2011). When analyzing an ABG it is important to record the volume of oxygen administered through oxygen therapy so that the effects of this can be evaluated (Gibson & Waters, 2017). Indications for undertaking an ABG include:

- Any unexpected deterioration in an ill patient.
- An acute exacerbation of a chronic chest condition or impaired respiratory effort particularly when the SpO2 falls below 92%.
- A decreased level of consciousness.
- A suspicion of sepsis.
- Any metabolic or electrolyte problem (Coleman & Morozowich, 2011).

The normal values for ABG results are presented in the box below.

> # Normal ABG parameters
>
> pH: 7.35–7.45
>
> PaO_2: 10–14 kPa*
>
> $PaCO_2$: 4.5–6 kPa*
>
> Base excess (BE): –2–+2 mmol/l
>
> HCO_3: 22–26 mmol/l
>
> Lactate: 1 mmol/l
>
> *1 kPa = 7.5 mmHg; P stands for the 'partial pressure of ...'

pH

Potential hydrogen (pH) measures acidity or alkalinity. Acids are chemicals that can release hydrogen ions (H+) whist alkaline can absorb hydrogen ions. The measure is in millimole per litre (mmol/l). Human blood is slightly alkaline ranging from pH 7.35 to 7.45. The main acid in blood, carbonic acid, is a weak acid (Gibson and Water, 2017).

pH is important because slight changes in it will affect enzyme activity. As has been discussed earlier, acidity reduces haemoglobin's affinity for oxygen, shifting the dissociation curve to the right – the Bohr effect. This will reduce myocardial contractility and thus cardiac output.

Acid base is affected by both respiratory and metabolic functions. The pH alone will not identify if the underlying cause is respiratory or metabolic. The body will attempt to maintain homeostasis especially regarding pH through compensation. That is, if there is say a metabolic acidosis, the body will stimulate an opposing abnormality such as a respiratory alkalosis to try and maintain a normal pH. The type of abnormality and the compensation can only be deter-mined through analysing the pH along with the respiratory and metabolic components.

Anaerobic respiration due to reduced tissue perfusion will result in the production of lactic acid. This can result in a life-threatening metabolic acidosis.

How to interpret an ABG

A systematic approach to ABG interpretation leads to easy interpretation. The five-step approach to ABG analysis provides one such approach (Cutler & Cutler, 2010):

- Step 1

Assess oxygenation. Is the patient hypoxic? What is the PaO_2 – how much oxygen was the patient on when the gas was taken?

- Step 2

Determine the status of the pH or Hydrogen Ion concentration. This is done by asking what is the pH and is the patient acidaemic or alkalaemic? If the pH is less than 7.35 (H+ > 45 nmol l-1) the patient is acidotic. If the pH is greater than 7.45 (H+ < 35 nmol l-1) the patient is alkalotic.

- Step 3

Determine the respiratory component. This is done by asking what is the $PaCO_2$? If the $PaCO_2$ is greater than 6.0 kPa (45 mmHg) the patient has a respiratory acidosis. If the $PaCO_2$ is less than 4.7 kPa (35 mmHg), the patient has a respiratory alkalosis.

- Step 4

Determine the metabolic component. In an ABG this is demonstrated through the HCO_3 and base excess results. This is done by asking: What is the HCO_3 and base excess?

   Bicarbonate is produced by the kidneys and liver and acts as the main buffer in plasma to maintain a normal pH. The normal range for bicarbonate is 22–26 mmol/l. If there are additional acids in the blood, the level of bicarbonate will fall as the bicarbonate ions are used to buffer the acids. If the HCO_3 is less than 22 mmol/l the patient has a metabolic acidosis. If the HCO_3 is greater than 26 mmol/l the patient has a metabolic alkalosis.

   A metabolic acidosis will also be represented by the base excess. The base excess is a derived figure indicating the number of moles of acid or base needed to return a litre of blood to a normal pH. If it is below –2 mEq/L the patient has a metabolic acidosis, whilst if it is above +2 mEq/L, they have a metabolic alkalosis.

- Step 5

Combine the information from the pH, $PaCO_2$ and the bicarbonate to determine the primary disturbance and whether there is any metabolic or respiratory compensation.

   Table 4.2 shows three examples of compensated and uncompensated ABG results.

Table 4.2   Examples of compensated and uncompensated ABG results

Compensated metabolic acidosis	Metabolic alkalosis	Uncompensated metabolic acidosis
pH 7.37	pH 7.55	pH 7.25
PaO_2 10.9 kPa	PaO_2 8.7 kPa	PaO_2 13 kPa
$PaCO_2$ 3.1 kPa	$PaCO_2$ 4.8 kPa	$PaCO_2$ 5.8 kPa
HCO_3 −21.6 mmol/l	HCO_3 −32 mmol/l	HCO_3 −12 mmol/l
BE −3.5 mEq/L	BE + 8 mEq/L	BE −10 mEq/L
SaO_2 99%	SaO_2 98%	SaO_2 95%
Lactate 0.5 mmol/l	Lactate 1 mmol/l	Lactate 4.7 mmol/l
This patient has a normal oxygen level because they are receiving 4l/min O_2 therapy. The Ph is normal because they are compensating through hyperventilating and 'blowing off' the CO_2. Overall, this patient has a slight metabolic acidosis, which has respiratory compensation.	This patient has a metabolic alkalosis. Ventilation is acceptable, the PaO_2 and $PaCO_2$ is adequate on 28% oxygen via non-invasive positive pressure ventilation (NIPPV). This patient was admitted with a community acquired left lower lobe pneumonia. This caused an initial respiratory acidosis, which initiated metabolic compensation to maintain homeostasis and a normal pH. The NIPPV removed the respiratory acidosis, however the metabolic compensation continues, resulting in the metabolic alkalosis.	This patient has a severe metabolic acidosis. The patient is ventilating adequately as the PaO_2 and $PaCO_2$ are acceptable, even though the patient is fully ventilated on 60% oxygen. However, the bicarbonate and base excess are very low, and lactate is high, indicating poor tissue perfusion and anaerobic respiration at cellular level.

PATHOPHYSIOLOGY – RESPIRATORY FAILURE

Respiratory failure is the inability to maintain adequate gas exchange and is characterised by abnormal arterial blood concentrations of oxygen and, in certain cases, carbon dioxide (British Thoracic Society (BTS), 2002). There are two types of respiratory failure – Type I and Type II.

Type I respiratory failure

Type I respiratory failure refers to hypoxaemia. This is the result of diseases that damage the lung tissues and results in difficulties with external respiration and the movement of oxygen from the alveoli into the circulation. This results in impaired gas diffusion across the alveolar–capillary membrane. There is a disturbance between the ventilation (gas) and the perfusion (the blood) and results in a significant shunt. This is referred to as a ventilation/perfusion mismatch and is abbreviated to V/Q mismatch.

The levels of carbon dioxide will initially remain normal or even lower as the patient will start to hyperventilate to compensate for the lack of oxygen. In Type I respiratory failure, the cells will enter anaerobic respiration. Here there will be an accumulation in lactic acid, which will result in a metabolic acidosis developing with associated hypoxaemia. This can result in multi-organ disfunction. The causes of Type I respiratory failure can be seen in the box below (BTS, 2002).

Common causes of Type I respiratory failure

Pulmonary (ventilation) causes

Atelectasis or collapse of the alveoli

Pneumonia, which is often the result of an infection that causes inflammation of the lung tissue

Acute Respiratory Distress Syndrome (ARDS)

Asthma

Pleural Effusion

An acute exacerbation of Chronic Obstructive Pulmonary Disease

Vascular (perfusion) causes

Pulmonary embolism

Pulmonary oedema, which is an accumulation of fluid in the lungs secondary to a reduced cardiac output

---

Type II respiratory failure

Type II respiratory failure relates to a raised circulating carbon dioxide level in the blood (hypercapnia) with or without hypoxaemia. This type of respiratory failure is related to reduced ventilation, that is the movement of air into and out of the airways and lungs (BTS, 2016).

Ultimately the person is unable to excrete the carbon dioxide and it accumulates in the circulation causing a respiratory acidosis, which again may lead to multi-organ dysfunction. If this becomes a chronic issue, the body responds by producing increased levels of buffers (namely bicarbonate) to compensate for this type of respiratory failure. This is seen particularly in patients with chronic obstructive pulmonary disease (COPD). This can then be exacerbated by an acute illness such as a chest infection (BTS, 2016).

If this happens, the patient will develop acute hypercapnic respiratory failure (AHRF), which results from an inability of the body to provide sufficient alveolar ventilation to maintain a normal $PaCO_2$. Hypoxaemia is usually mild and easily corrected. Conventionally, a pH less than 7.35 and a $PaCO_2$ greater than 6.5 kPa define acute respiratory acidosis (BTS, 2016). The causes of Type II respiratory failure can be seen below.

Common causes of Type II respiratory failure

Respiratory depression by opiate overdose or a traumatic brain injury

Acute chest infection, asthma or pneumonia

Spinal injury

Acute neuromuscular disease such as myasthenia gravis or Guillain-Barre syndrome

Pneumothorax or haemothorax

Airway obstruction

Consider the following case study:

Tom is a 37 year old primary school teacher. Over the past week a number of children have been coughing and spluttering within his classroom. Tom has taken himself to the doctors today as he has had a productive cough over the past few days and is feeling hot and flushed. He has had very little sleep over the past three nights and is feeling physically exhausted.

On examination the doctor finds:

Airway: Tom's airway is patent. He is able to converse in short clipped sentences. The base of his lungs sounds dull and there is little air entry to this area.

Breathing: Tom's respiratory rate is 28 breaths per minute. Tom is using his accessory muscles. Tom's saturations are 94% and he is coughing up purulent sputum, which the doctor sends for M,C &S.

Circulation: Tom's heart rate is 127 beats per minute, bounding strong pulse. His blood pressure is 110/70 mmHg. Tom feels warm and flushed and his temperature is 38.5⁰. His capillary refill time is 2 seconds. Tom last passed urine two hours ago, however there wasn't very much there, and it was dark in colour.

(Continued)

Disability: Tom is not a diabetic and his blood sugar levels are fine. He is complaining of right shoulder pain. He is alert and orientated.

Exposure: There are no signs of a rash on Tom. He has a dry mouth and skin.

The doctor took some blood tests. One of these was an arterial blood gas taken on air. The results of this were:

pH 7.35

PaO_2 7.2 kPa

$PaCO_2$ 4.2 kPa

HCO_3 –21 mmol/l

Lactate 2 mmol/l

BE –3

SaO_2 92%

The doctor diagnosed a lower respiratory tract infection and prescribed a course of oral amoxicillin.

What type of respiratory failure does Tom have?

Explain the underlying pathophysiology to Tom's clinical condition.

Using a systematic approach, analyse Tom's arterial blood gas result.

SUMMARY

This chapter has presented the anatomy and physiology of the respiratory system. Normal external, internal and cellular respiration have been explored. A systematic approach to arterial blood gas analysis has been presented and the underlying pathophysiology of respiratory failure considered. The management of Type I and Type II respiratory failure will be addressed in the following chapter.

REFERENCES

British Thoracic Society (BTS) (2002) *Guideline on Non-invasive Ventilation in Acute Respiratory Failure.* London: BTS.

British Thoracic Society (BTS) (2016) *BTS Guidelines for the Ventilatory Management of Acute Hypercapnic Respiratory Failure*. London: BTS.

Clancy, J. & McVicar, A. (2009) *Physiology and Anatomy for Nurses and Healthcare Practitioners: A Homeostatic Approach* (3rd ed.). London: Hodder Arnold.

Coleman, M. D. & Morozowich, S. T. (2011) Blood gas and acid base analysis. In J. Duke, *Anaesthesia Secrets* (4th ed.) (pp. 24–30). Philadelphia: Mosby.

Cook, N., Shepherd, A. & Boore, J. (2021) *Essentials of Anatomy and Physiology in Nursing Practice* (2nd ed.). London: SAGE.

Credland, N. (2017) In Gibson, V. and Waters, D. *Respiratory Care*. London. Taylor Francis Group

Cutler, L. & Cutler, J. (2010) *Critical Care Nursing Made Incredibly Easy*. London: Lippincott Williams and Wilkins.

Gibson, V. and Waters D. (2017) *Respiratory Care*. London. Taylor Francis Group.

McLafferty, E., Johnstone, C., Hendry, C. & Farley, A. (2013a) Respiratory system part 1: Pulmonary ventilation. *Nursing Standard*, 27 (22), 40–47.

McLafferty, E., Johnstone, C., Hendry, C. & Farley, A. (2013b) Respiratory system part 2: Gaseous exchange. *Nursing Standard*, 27 (23), 35–42.

Peate, I. (2018) Anatomy and physiology 10. The respiratory system. *British Journal of Healthcare Assistants* 12 (4).

Tortora, G. J. & Derrickson, B. H. (2017) *Principles of Anatomy and Physiology* (15th ed.). New York: Wiley.

5

PATIENT-CENTRED APPROACHES TO BREATHING: APPLICATION TO PRACTICE

SARAH MCGLOIN

Chapter learning outcomes

By the end of this chapter you will be able to:

1. Assess a patient using the ABCDE approach.
2. Identify the signs and symptoms of an individual who is experiencing difficulties breathing.
3. Recognise when and how to escalate care.
4. Plan and implement evidence-based care for patients experiencing difficulties breathing.
5. Understand the underlying pathophysiology to those experiencing difficulties breathing.

Key words

- ABCDE assessment
- Type I respiratory failure
- Type II respiratory failure
- Community acquired pneumonia
- Chronic obstructive pulmonary disease
- Asthma
- Pneumothorax
- Sepsis Six

INTRODUCTION

This chapter will present three case studies of patients who are experiencing difficulties with their respiratory system. For each case study, an initial assessment will take place to identify and prioritise the patient's key problems. The underlying pathophysiology will then be explored followed by evidence-based interventions and management strategies for each of the four case studies. The case studies will focus on: community acquired pneumonia; chronic obstructive pulmonary disease; asthma; and pneumothorax.

Activity 5.1

Read the following case study. What type of respiratory failure does Kerry have?

CASE STUDY 5.1: COMMUNITY ACQUIRED PNEUMONIA – KERRY ANDERSON

Case study 5.1 takes a look at a patient with a community acquired pneumonia (CAP). This is a cause of Type I respiratory failure, where there is acute hypoxaemia with a normal circulating arterial carbon dioxide level. Type I respiratory failure is caused by an acute respiratory event such as CAP. Up to 1% of adults within the UK will develop a CAP annually (NICE, 2014). Of these, 22–44% will be admitted to hospital where the mortality rate is between 5 and 14% (NICE, 2014). A summary of Kerry's observations on admission are presented below.

Box 5.1 Kerry's initial assessment

Kerry Anderson (35) has been admitted to the medical assessment unit (MAU) via her family doctor with a week long history of a productive cough, which gets worse at night. Kerry is normally fit and healthy, visiting the gym three times a week. She weighs 90 kg. On admission, Kerry's observations were:

Airway

- Kerry was able to speak in short clipped sentences but looked exhausted doing so. She was leaning forward onto her arms, which were extended over the bedtable

(Continued)

- Productive cough with purulent sputum
- Crackles on oscillation

Breathing

- Respiratory rate: 32 breaths per minute (bpm)
- Oxygen saturation levels: 85% on air
- Chest X-ray demonstrated left lower lobe basal collapse indicating a left lower lobe pneumonia

Circulation

- Blood pressure: 85/68 mmHg
- Heart rate: 121 beats per minute
- Temperature: 38.9° C
- Urine output: 22, 15 and 7 mls/hour over the past three hours
- Capillary refill time (CRT): 2 seconds

Disability

- Confused on ACVPU; disorientated to time and place
- Pain score 2/3 with complaints of right shoulder pain and pain on inspiration
- Blood sugar: 6.7 mmol/l

Exposure

- Pressure areas intact
- Lips were dry and cracked

Community acquired pneumonia

Kerry's chest X-ray demonstrated a left lower lobe CAP. This is the result of an infection of lung tissue obtained outside any hospital or healthcare setting (NICE, 2014). Whilst a chest X-ray provides the gold standard for diagnosis, other signs and symptoms will include:

- Dyspnoea
- Tachypnoea
- Fatigue
- Symptoms of acute lower respiratory tract illness such as cough and one other lower respiratory tract symptom

- New focal chest sounds on examination such as crackles (indicating fluid on the lungs)
- At least one systemic feature such as:
  - ○ Pyrexia greater than 38°C
  - ○ Shivers, chills or night sweats
  - ○ Aches and pains especially pleuritic chest pain
- No other explanation for acute illness, which is treated as CAP with antibiotics

Other diagnostic factors include:

- Symptoms consistent with a lower acute respiratory tract infection associated with new radiographic shadowing for which there is no other explanation
- The illness is the primary reason for admission

Activity 5.2

Describe the underlying pathophysiology of Kerry's condition.

Pathophysiology

Pneumonia relates to the presence of fluid within the alveoli (Gibson and Waters, 2017). CAP develops when the innate immune system within the respiratory tract and lungs becomes overwhelmed by inhaled pathogens (BMJ, 2020). The pathogens from the upper airways enter the lower respiratory tract and the lungs where they cause pneumonia. Pneumonia is the result of infection by bacteria, the main one being Streptococcus pneumonia, a gram-positive organism (Morgan & Glossop, 2016). Other infections that can cause pneumonia include 'atypical' bacteria such as Legionella pneumophilia, the influenza virus, fungi or chemical agents such as aspiration pneumonia (Gibson and Waters, 2017)). The infection Kerry has is a community acquired streptococcus pneumonia. The signs and symptoms of pneumonia are the result of the effects of the pathogen on the lung parenchyma and neighbouring tissues. There are four stages to developing CAP.

Stage one is the congestion stage. This is the early acute inflammatory response by the pro-inflammatory mediators in the alveoli. Here the infected alveoli become red and oedematous as a result of increased capillary permeability in the region. Fluid moves from the capillary into the alveoli. This stage lasts from between 24 and 48 hours, during which the alveoli become filled with fluid and bacteria referred to as exudate. It is this fluid that becomes evident on the chest X-ray. This exudate contains neutrophils, lymphocytes and fibrin and fills the alveoli sacs.

At the same time, the pulmonary capillaries become congested. This all results in a V/Q mismatch and a shunt with deoxygenated blood being circulated. As a compensatory mechanism, the heart rate increases in an attempt to increase the cardiac output and flow of blood through the lungs. This inflammation results in the pleuritic pain Kerry is experiencing.

The second stage is the hepatisation stage. This lasts for 2 to 4 days and is characterised by a reddening of the affected lobes, which also lose their compliance meaning the alveoli become stiff and hard and difficult to ventilate. The alveoli also become red at this stage as red blood cells leak from the capillaries into the lung parenchyma. At this point, Kerry's lungs will become hyperaemic where the capillaries are engorged with blood and the fibrin fill the alveoli (Gibson, 2015). This all results in congestion within the capillaries and alveoli, which causes pulmonary hypertension. This then forces more fluid out of the capillaries into the alveoli and they become even more oedematous, resulting in pulmonary oedema. At this point, there is also a slight increase in body temperature.

The third stage is grey hepatisation where the affected alveoli become dry, firm and grey as a result of the lysed red blood cells. White blood cells including leucocytes and macrophages become noticeable at this stage and the pathogens' presence should start to decrease as these white blood cells work to remove them. The pressure from the exudate within the collapsed alveoli causes compression of the pulmonary capillaries. This results in a continuing V/Q mismatch. The respiratory rate increases to try and compensate for this.

Finally, there is the resolution phase. Enzymes act within the alveoli and break down the fibrous clots sitting within the alveoli. Ventilation of the lungs is restored. During this stage a large number of macrophages enter the alveoli and phagocytose the leukocytes. There is a reduction of fluid and cellular exudate as the fluid is expectorated up and out of the airway or reabsorbed through the lymphatic system. The parenchyma of the lungs should be restored to normal within three weeks.

Activity 5.3

Discuss the management plan for Kerry based upon the National Drivers and evidence base.

Management of community acquired pneumonia

Management of CAP in the UK is driven by two clinical drivers: The NICE CG 191 *Pneumonia in adults: Diagnosis and management* (NICE, 2014 updated in 2019) and the *Guidelines for the management of community acquired pneumonia in adults update* (BTS, 2009).

Assessment

Following on from the initial set of observations that were carried out, a number of assessment strategies were carried out as soon as Kerry was admitted to assess her condition. These were:

- National Early Warning Score (2) (Royal College of Physicians [RCP], 2017)
- Sepsis Six (NICE, 2017a; Sepsis Trust, 2019)
- CURB65 score (NICE, 2014)

On admission to MAU, a NEWS2 score was firstly completed. This found Kerry had a very high NEWS2 score of 15, which necessitated immediate referral to an emergency response team such as the critical care outreach team (RCP, 2017). This was because Kerry was at great risk of rapid deterioration.

Whilst the admitting nurse caring for Kerry was contacting the critical care outreach team, she asked another nurse to implement the Sepsis Six bundle (NICE, 2017a; Sepsis Trust, 2019). This was done concurrently with no delay as the admitting nurse had a high suspicion that Kerry had developed sepsis. In line with the National Confidential Enquiry into Patient Outcome and Death (NCEPOD) report *Just Say Sepsis* (NCEPOD, 2015), the nurse understood to implement the Sepsis Six bundle with immediate effect.

Box 5.2 Sepsis Six

Three in:

1. Oxygen therapy
2. Administering broad spectrum antibiotics
3. Administering IV fluids

Three out:

4. Measuring lactate
5. Taking blood cultures and sending them off for MC and S analysis
6. Measuring hourly urine output, which should be at 0.5 ml/kg/hour

---

Applying the Sepsis Six bundle to Kerry meant she:

1. Was commenced on oxygen therapy through a non-rebreathe oxygen mask at 15l/min with the aim of keeping her SaO_2 above 94% (NICE, 2017a).

2. Had blood cultures taken and sent off for MC and S analysis.
3. Had broad spectrum antibiotics administered.
4. Had her serum lactate measured. If it was above 4 mmol/l, referral to critical care outreach was necessary.
5. Had IV fluids (crystalloids) administered. Kerry had a fluid bolus of 500 mls of crystalloid. The fluid continued not exceeding 30 mls/kg.
6. Had her hourly urine output recorded, which should be at 0.5 ml/kg/hour and in Kerry's case was 45 mls/hr.

In addition to the Sepsis Six, a catheter stream urine (CSU) and sputum samples were obtained and sent for MC&S. Because there was a high suspicion that Kerry had a CAP, the next stage was to diagnose this through a CURB65 score (NICE, 2014). This indicated how severe Kerry's CAP was. The CURB65 criteria are presented in Box 5.3.

Kerry scored a 2 on the CURB65 and so was at intermediate risk of death at 3–15% mortality risk. Based on this assessment and in line with the NICE (2014) guidelines, the decision was made to admit Kerry via the MAU to a high dependency unit where Kerry could receive close observation. This was because Kerry was at extreme risk of sudden deterioration.

Box 5.3 The CURB65 criteria

CURB65 score for mortality risk assessment in hospital

CURB65 score is calculated by giving 1 point for each of the following prognostic features:

- Confusion (abbreviated Mental Test score 8 or less, or new disorientation in person, place or time)
- Raised blood urea nitrogen (over 7 mmol/l)
- Raised respiratory rate (30 breaths per minute or more)
- Low blood pressure (diastolic 60 mmHg or less, or systolic less than 90 mmHg)
- Age 65 years or more

Patients are stratified for risk of death as follows:

- 0 or 1: low risk (less than 3% mortality risk)
- 2: intermediate risk (3–15% mortality risk)
- 3 to 5: high risk (more than 15% mortality risk)

Source: NICE, 2014

Once the MC&S results were back, Kerry was treated with the appropriate antibiotic. The NICE CG (2014) recommends a 7–10 day course of antibiotics to manage moderate to severe CAP such as Kerry had.

Ongoing management

The issue with Kerry's CAP was to ensure an adequate delivery of oxygen to the tissues to enable cellular respiration to occur. Without adequate tissue perfusion, the tissues will become under perfused and the cells will enter anaerobic respiration. A by-product of this is lactic acid. Therefore, through measuring a patient's lactate in conjunction with other parameters such as respiratory rate, blood pressure and urine output, it is possible to say if the tissue perfusion is adequate. To help with this assessment an ABG is helpful. Kerry had an ABG sample taken when she was in the MAU receiving 15l/min oxygen therapy. The results are presented in Box 5.4

Box 5.4 Arterial blood gas result

pH 7.32

PaO_2 9.5 kPa

$PaCO_2$ 4.5 kPa

HCO_3 –24 mmol/l

Lactate 4.7 mmol/l

BE –9.2

SaO_2 95%

The ABG was analysed using the five step approach as presented in Chapter 4 (Cutler & Cutler, 2010).

Oxygenation was seen to be acceptable, however Kerry was on 15l/min. The pH was low, indicating an acidosis. The carbon dioxide was also acceptable although Kerry's respiratory rate remained elevated at 22 breaths per minute when the sample was taken. The bicarbonate and base excess readings were low, indicating that the body's buffers were working hard to maintain homeostasis. The lactate was high demonstrating reduced tissue perfusion and the presence of anaerobic respiration. This ABG result demonstrates that Kerry has an uncompensated metabolic acidosis, secondary to sepsis with a CAP as the source of origin. The oxygen dissociation curve will have shifted to the right in relation to the Bohr effect as a result of the acidosis and high temperature. This combined with the V/Q mismatch caused by the left lower lobe basal collapse means that there is relative hypoxaemia and reduced tissue perfusion.

To manage this situation, Kerry required further fluid therapy to enhance her peripheral tissue perfusion. Strategies should also be implemented to manage her V/Q mismatch and to try and reduce the forced inspired oxygen concentration (FiO_2) she was receiving. High FiO_2 for prolonged periods of time are found to cause oxygen toxicity and exacerbate inflammation of the lung parenchyma through the release of free radicals. Additionally, Kerry was still receiving non-humidified oxygen therapy. This can lead to the airways drying out, making it difficult to clear secretions that could exacerbate an intra-pulmonary shunt.

On admission to the HDU, Kerry remained on 15l/min of oxygen via a non-rebreathe bag. She received two boluses of 500 mls Hartmann's solution and had a litre of maintenance fluid (Hartmann's solution) running at 125 mls/hour. Kerry had received a dose of dual broad spectrum antibiotics in line with the NICE CG191 (NICE, 2014) including amoxicillin and a macrolide. She had been catheterised and an urometer was in situ. Kerry had also received paracetamol as both antipyretic therapy and analgesia. Kerry's observations were as presented in Box 5.5.

Box 5.5 Kerry's observations following commencement of Sepsis Six

Airway

- Patent. Kerry was able to speak in short sentences. She was no longer slumped over the bedtable
- Chest sounds still crackles

Breathing

- Respiratory rate: 22 bpm
- SaO_2: 94%
- Dry cough

Circulation

- Blood pressure: 112/72 mmHg
- Heart rate: 104 beats per minute
- Temperature: 37.9° C

(Continued)

- Urine output: 45 mls/hour
- Capillary refill time (CRT): 2 seconds

Disability

- A on ACVPU
- Pain score 1/3
- Blood sugar: 6.4 mmol/l

Exposure

- Pressure areas intact
- Lips less dry

Following her fluid resuscitation, Kerry's ABG results were now as presented in Box 5.6

Box 5.6 Arterial blood gas result

pH 7.34

PaO_2 9.7 kPa

$PaCO_2$ 4.7 kPa

HCO_3 – 25 mmol/l

Lactate 2.9 mmol/l

BE –6.5

SaO_2 95%

This demonstrates that Kerry still has a metabolic acidosis but that it is improving with the fluid and oxygen therapy.

Activity 5.4

Analyse the arterial blood gas result. What does it show?

Management on the HDU

Airway and breathing

Kerry's oxygen therapy needs to be changed from a non-rebreathe bag to a venturi mask. A venturi mask is a fixed performance oxygen mask, which entrains air and oxygen through a venturi valve and mixes them together to deliver a fixed amount of inspired oxygen. This system can also be attached to a humidifier, which prevents the airways from drying out. This means a fixed FiO_2 can be delivered and titrated to the ABG or SaO_2 results.

Kerry's V/Q mismatch may also be addressed through patient positioning. Kerry's chest X-ray demonstrates a left lower lobe pneumonia. Therefore, to reduce her V/Q mismatch, placing Kerry on her right hand side (or 'good lung down') can enhance the external respiration and movement of gases. This is because the dependent lung (the part of the lungs that is best ventilated) is placed next to the circulation. By positioning Kerry with her good lung down, this also enables access for chest physiotherapy to the poor lung. Chest X-rays will help determine the dependent lung thus facilitating best positioning.

Circulation

Kerry needs to receive fluid therapy to ensure her blood pressure and cardiac output remain acceptable. The administration of the antibiotics will treat the underlying cause, which is the CAP. This should eventually reduce the capillary permeability as the infection recedes, enabling stage four of the CAP process to be reached. Urine output needs to be monitored hourly to ensure Kerry does not develop an Acute Kidney Injury. Her temperature needs to be taken to monitor her basal metabolic rate and response to infection. Kerry's capillary refill time also needs to be monitored as an indication of peripheral tissue perfusion. A delayed CRT coupled with a raised lactate will indicate peripheral vasoconstriction and reduced tissue perfusion at the peripheries. This is a sign that the patient requires additional fluid resuscitation.

Disability

ACVPU needs to be undertaken within the NEWS2 scoring. This will demonstrate how effective Kerry's cerebral perfusion is. Kerry requires regular assessment for pleuritic pain, which again will improve once the infection recedes. Blood sugar levels need to be monitored to evaluate the sympathetic nervous system response to this acute illness. In times of physiological stress such as during an infection, the SNS will mobilise glucose through glycogenolysis to ensure there is adequate glucose available for cellular respiration.

Exposure

At all times Kerry's pressure areas should be assessed. With her reduced mobility and nutrition, Kerry is at risk of developing pressure sores. Kerry should be encouraged to mobilise as early as possible, to prevent further chest consolidation due to reduced mobility and pressure sores developing.

Kerry should remain on regular observations using the NEWS2 assessment strategy. Any deterioration in her condition should be escalated using the Situation Background Assessment and Recommendation (SBAR) strategy to the critical care outreach team. Kerry can be discharged when she has responded to treatment and been stable. Kerry will not be able to be discharged if she has in the past 24 hours had two or more of the following:

- Temperature higher than 37.5°C
- Respiratory rate 24 bpm or more
- Tachycardia over 100 bpm
- Systolic blood pressure of 90 mmHg or less
- Oxygen saturation below 90% on room air
- Altered mental status
- Inability to eat without assistance

Discharge should also be delayed for patients with CAP if their temperature is higher than 37.5°C.

Activity 5.5

Read the following case study. Explain what COPD actually is.

CASE STUDY 5.2: CHRONIC OBSTRUCTIVE PULMONARY DISEASE – WINNIE ETHEREDGE

Case study 5.2 focuses on Winnie Etheredge who has been diagnosed with chronic obstructive pulmonary disease (COPD). COPD is an umbrella term used to describe conditions including chronic bronchitis and emphysema. Currently 1.2 million people are diagnosed with COPD, although this could actually be up to 3.6 million (NICE, 2018). Most recent data shows that a total of 14,760 people died from COPD in England and Wales in 2015 (NHS Digital, 2018) and it is said that one person dies from COPD every 20 minutes in England (NHS England, 2012). To enhance the care of patients with COPD, NHS England (2018) published the *NHS RightCare Pathway for COPD*. A summary of Winnie's observations on admission are presented in Box 5.7.

Chronic Obstructive Pulmonary Disease

Winnie has been admitted with an acute exacerbation of her COPD. A severe exacerbation of COPD will be demonstrated through:

- Acute confusion
- Reduced ability to carry out activities of daily living
- Shortness of breath and tachypnoea
- Pursed lip breathing
- Use of accessory respiratory muscles whilst at rest
- Peripheral oedema
- Newly onset cyanosis

Red flag signs and symptoms for COPD include:

- Haemoptysis
- Breathlessness
- Wheezing
- Drowsiness or agitation
- Fever
- Chest pain (Mitchell, 2015)

Pathophysiology

> ## Activity 5.6
>
> Describe the underlying pathophysiology of Winnie's condition.

COPD involves an obstruction to airflow through the airway and cigarette smoke is by far the strongest risk factor (Hooper et al., 2012) with occupation and air pollution also responsible (Baraldo et al., 2012). This obstruction makes ventilation – the movement of air into and out of the lungs – more difficult and is the result of chronic, irreversible inflammation of the airways, lung parenchyma, alveoli and pulmonary vasculature. The airways become narrowed and remodelled with an increased number of goblet cells, which produce thick secretions (Peate & Dutton, 2021). There is also an enlargement of the mucous-secreting glands of the central airways. Lung tissue becomes stiff with poor compliance due to a loss in the elastic recoil of lung tissue. There are also vascular bed changes resulting in pulmonary hypertension (BMJ Best Practice, 2021).

Bronchoconstriction

Airways become narrowed in COPD due to the contraction of smooth bronchial tissue, inflammation and mucous production (Mitchell, 2015). This results in the wheeze airway sound associated with a patient with COPD. This is the result of turbulent airflow through narrowed airways (see Figure 5.1).

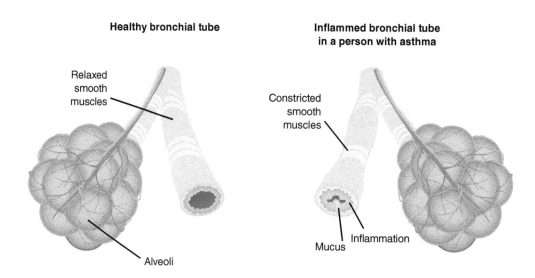

Figure 5.1   Bronchoconstriction

Mucous hypersecretion

Cilia dysfunction and excessive mucous secretion result in a productive cough. This can result in up to 100 ml of mucus being produced each day (Peate & Dutton, 2021). This occurs due to cigarette smoke causing direct injury to the respiratory epithelium, which lines the respiratory tree. Cigarette smoke causes the respiration mucosa to become infiltrated by inflammatory cells, which then cause an increase in the production of mucus. The tissue is unable to repair itself from this inflammation and the airways become thick and poorly compliant. Not only does smoking increase mucus secretion, but dehydration and oxygen therapy can also contribute as well.

This increased sputum production is the result of structural changes in the airway alongside a chronic inflammatory response with the loss of elastic recoil of bronchial tissue, which causes the airways to narrow and close early during expiration. The mucus secreting cells multiply and thus increase the viscosity and volume of mucus secretion. The lumen of the airway then becomes occluded by mucus plugs from an excess of inflammatory exudate (Kauffman, 2011). Purulent secretions are the result of degenerating white blood cells whilst rusty secretions are a sign of pneumonia.

Cough

When irritant receptors within the airway are stimulated by either chemicals (smoke), inflammation (histamine) or foreign bodies, a cough is stimulated as a protective mechanism. A chronic, productive cough however due to COPD is the result of increased mucosal secretion from the goblet cells in the bronchial wall in response to chronic inflammation. Constant coughing can also cause the patient to feel constantly fatigued.

Dyspnoea and tachypnoea

A very common symptom of acute or chronic COPD is shortness of breath. This results when the demand for gas to be moved into and out of the airways is out of proportion to the individual's ability to meet that demand. This results in laboured breathing, which is uncomfortable and tiring for the patient.

Dyspnoea can be regarded to be the sixth vital sign in a patient with COPD (Hill Bailey et al., 2013). The greater the respiratory effort for minimal gain, the worse the breathlessness is for a patient. A normal respiratory rate is regarded to sit between 12–20 breaths per minute. Anything over 20bpm is referred to as tachypnoea. There are a number of causes for this including pyrexia and COPD.

COPD also increases the work of breathing, which is 10–12 times greater in those with COPD. The work of breathing refers to the amount of energy required to move air into and out of the lungs. Inspiration uses energy. As patients with COPD have poor lung compliance, it takes more energy for the patient to inspire and expand their lungs and airways. Therefore the patient with COPD has to work harder to ventilate their lungs.

To help ventilate the lungs, the patient will make use of their accessory muscles. Under normal conditions as presented in Chapter 4, the diaphragm is the main respiratory muscle. Paradoxical breathing – which is the opposite of normal chest movement during inspiration and expiration – indicates respiratory fatigue. Then accessory muscles are recruited to increase the respiratory rate. Also to help ventilate their lungs, patients with COPD adopt forced breathing (or pursed lip breathing). During this, more energy is required for the patient to breathe and they start to use their accessory muscles. These include the abdominal muscles, sternocleido-mastoid, scalene and trapezius.

Respiratory failure in COPD

As has previously been discussed in Chapter 4, respiratory failure is the result of poor gas exchange and an increased work of breathing. Type II respiratory failure is associated with COPD. Here there is hypoxaemia combined with a raised criterial carbon dioxide level. This happens when ventilation is so poor it cannot excrete the CO_2 from the body.

Altered gas exchange in COPD

Gas exchange at the alveoli in some patients with COPD becomes altered due to hypoxic pulmonary vasoconstriction. This happens because the body is trying to reduce a ventilation/perfusion mismatch. To do this, the arteries around poorly ventilated alveoli constrict and the circulation is diverted to the alveoli, which are ventilated and full of gas. Over time, this results in pulmonary artery constriction, which can also be called 'pulmonary hypertension'. This will result in shortness of breath on exertion, palpitations, chest pain and syncope (Ward et al., 2015). If this is left to develop, chronic pulmonary hypertension results in the thickening of the pulmonary vessels causing abnormality in the route of blood vessels between the heart and the lungs.

Long term hypoxic vaso-constriction in COPD patients may lead to pulmonary hypertension or cor pulmonale. This can result in right sided heart failure developing and is the result of long term low oxygen levels causing narrowing of the pulmonary blood vessels. This causes a backflow to the heart. The right ventricle is unable to cope with this backflow and this can result in ankle and sacral oedema and ascites.

Hypercapnia and hypoxia in COPD

Carbon dioxide retention in COPD causes a respiratory acidosis. This is detected by the chemoreceptors in the medulla oblongata, which in turn inform the respiratory centre to increase the rate and depth of breathing.

Due to the chronic nature of their disease, patients with COPD often have a raised $PaCO_2$ level; however their body compensates through metabolic processes to maintain a normal pH and thus homeostasis. One quarter of patients with an acute exacerbation of their COPD are at risk of carbon dioxide retention if they are given very high doses of oxygen and this can reduce their respiratory drive. However, this is very rare and if a patient with COPD is hypoxic, the BTS oxygen therapy guidelines (2017) state that they must receive oxygen therapy at a rate to maintain their oxygen saturations between 88% and 92%. An arterial blood gas will provide the most reliable clinical picture on which to manage oxygen therapy for this type of patient.

An elevated CO_2 can also increase cardiac output in an attempt to enhance tissue perfusion. This can cause a bounding pulse, vasodilation and headaches from a raised cerebral blood flow. If the CO_2 becomes too high, patients can experience decreased levels of consciousness, which can deteriorate into coma.

Box 5.7 Winnie's initial assessment

Winnie Etheredge (82) was housebound and living on her own with social care support. Winnie's medical history included reduced mobility, hypertension and Type II diabetes. Winnie was obese and weighed 140 kg. She has just been admitted to the ward off her legs and unable to cope. It was found that she has Type II respiratory failure with an infective exacerbation of her COPD.

Airway

- Winnie was breathless but she was able to speak in short clipped sentences but looked exhausted doing so
- Productive cough with purulent sputum

Breathing

- Respiratory rate: 28 breaths per minute (bpm)
- Oxygen saturations were 82% on air. They are normally 91% on air
- Winnie was breathing through pursed lips. She had shallow breaths
- Chest expansion was equal on both sides
- Dull percussion to the mid zones of both her lungs and poor air entry was apparent to these areas as well as the bases
- Chest X-ray demonstrated bilateral basal collapse

Circulation

- Blood pressure: 89/67 mmHg
- Heart rate: 127 beats per minute
- Temperature: 37.9° C
- Urine output: 30, 27 and 14 mls/hour over the past three hours
- Capillary refill time (CRT): 2 seconds and she appeared vasodilated

Disability

- Winnie was excessively sleepy so V on the ACVPU
- Blood sugar: 9.8 mmol/l

(Continued)

Exposure

- Pressure areas intact
- Lips were dry and cracked

Management of an acute exacerbation of COPD

Management of COPD in the UK is driven by the NICE *NG 115 Chronic Obstructive Airways Disease in over 16s: Diagnosis and management.*

Activity 5.7

Discuss the management plan for Winnie based upon the National Drivers and evidence base.

Airway and breathing

Having assessed Winnie's airway as being patent, the first intervention she received was 28% oxygen therapy via a venturi mask (BTS, 2017). Her oxygen saturations improved only slightly to 84%. Winnie's saturations were monitored continuously, as was her respiratory rate. An arterial blood gas was then taken. The results of this are presented in Box 5.8.

Box 5.8 Arterial blood gas result

pH 7.31

PaO_2 6.7 kPa

$PaCO_2$ 8.7 kPa

HCO_3 – 29 mmol/l

Lactate 2 mmol/l

BE –2.0

SaO_2 84%

Activity 5.8

Analyse the arterial blood gas result. What does it show?

To enhance Winnie's oxygenation and to support her breathing and prevent her becoming exhausted, it was decided to move Winnie to a respiratory unit where she was commenced on Non Invasive Positive Pressure Ventilation (NIPPV) (BTS, 2016).

Non-invasive positive pressure ventilation (NIPPV)

Non-invasive positive pressure ventilation (NPPIV) is an umbrella term for 'the provision of ventilatory support through the patient's upper airway using a mask or similar device' (RCP/BTS/ICS, 2008). NIPPV can be either Continuous positive airways pressure (CPAP) or Bilevel positive airway pressure (BiPAP). NIPPV treatments aim to decrease the work of breathing and prevent patients becoming exhausted, increase tidal volume and decrease respiratory rate (BTS, 2008).

CPAP is indicated for patients with Type I respiratory failure or cardiogenic pulmonary oedema, whereas BiPAP is indicated for Type II respiratory failure but can also be used in specialist areas such as the intensive care unit (ICU) for weaning from invasive ventilation. NIPPV is generally contraindicated in patients with asthma and those patients who do not respond early in treatment (BTS, 2018).

NIPPV should be considered in all patients with an acute exacerbation of COPD and a respiratory acidosis having received controlled oxygen therapy for no more than one hour (BTS, 2018). As Winnie fell into this category, and had Type II respiratory failure, the plan was to give her non-invasive ventilation in the form of BiPAP. Here there would be an inspiratory positive airway pressure (IPAP) given as Winnie took a breath and a small amount of gas left in the lower airways at the end of her breath – Expiratory Positive Airway Pressure (EPAP). The rationale for this is that it makes it easier for Winnie to take the next breath in.

Winnie was sat leaning forward and started on NIPPIV. The therapy was delivered via a full-face mask for the first 24 hours. Initially Winnie had an inspiratory positive airway pressure (IPAP) of 10 cms H_2O and expiratory positive airway pressure (EPAP) of 4–5 cms H_2O. Whilst these levels allowed Winnie to become acclimatised to the NIPPV machine, an ABG taken two hours after the treatment had commenced (BTS, 2016), demonstrating the NIPPV had failed to significantly improve her gas exchange.

The IPAP was therefore gradually increased by 2–5 cm increments at a rate of approximately 5 cms H_2O each 10 minutes, all the time ensuring Winnie could tolerate these increases.

This happened until a therapeutic IPAP of 20 cms H_2O was achieved. A 4–5 cms EPAP setting reduces CO_2 re-breathing and assists triggering of the ventilator when using BiPAP.

Oxygen was entrained into the NIPPV machine and adjusted to maintain the target saturation, of 88–92% (BTS, 2016) for Winnie.

Having initially addressed Winnie's breathing, the team decided to administer inhaled therapy using a nebuliser as Winnie was quite weak and had difficulty using an inhaler. The inhaled therapy involved a salbutamol, which is used for immediate relief of bronchoconstriction. Winnie was also prescribed Ipratropium Bromide of 250–500 micrograms 3–4 times a day. This can be used for short-term relief in mild COPD for patients who are not using a long-acting antimuscarinic drug. Its maximal effect occurs 30–60 minutes after use; its duration of action is 3 to 6 hours and bronchodilation can usually be maintained with treatment three times a day.

Nebulisers can be driven by compressed air or oxygen. They create a mist of drug particles that are inhaled via a facemask or mouthpiece. It was felt that this was more appropriate for Winnie as with an inhaler, not only did she lack the strength to press the device, a substantial proportion of the drug was also deposited in her oropharynx meaning she did not receive the full amount. When Winnie was discharged home, she had a spacer device that was attached to a metered dose inhaler. This helps patients such as Winnie with their technique as the spacer avoids problems in coordinating the timing of inhaler actuation and inhalation. The rate of delivery of the spray into the mouth is slowed, which results in less drug being deposited in the oropharynx and more in the lower airways. If used correctly, a metered dose inhaler with spacer is at least as effective as any other device for delivering inhaled drugs.

Further to the inhaled therapy, Winnie was also prescribed 30 mg oral prednisolone for seven days initially. The nebulisers reduced the bronchoconstriction and improved her expiratory wheeze. The corticosteroids also reduced the inflammation present in her airways. Winnie's peak flow was recorded daily to monitor recovery from her acute exacerbation of her COPD.

A sputum sample was sent for MC&S, and blood cultures were also taken as Winnie had a pyrexia (NICE, 2017a). As Winnie was showing red flags for sepsis, she was started on the Sepsis Six (Sepsis Trust, 2019) care bundle, which included broad spectrum antibiotics being prescribed. Once the results of the sputum sample were back, these were changed to an antibiotic suitable to treat the bacterial infection.

Circulation

Winnie's ECG showed nothing abnormal other than a sinus tachycardia. Again, in response to this being a red flag for sepsis, Winnie was given a 500 ml crystalloid fluid bolus. Her urine output was continuously monitored. Further fluid boluses were given until her urine output returned to 0.5 ml/kg/hr. Winnie was prescribed paracetamol 1 g every six hours to reduce her temperature and the additional oxygen demand this caused. In line with the guidelines (NICE, 2018), a full blood count, and urea and electrolytes blood samples were taken.

Disability

Winnie's ACVPU was recorded hourly and as her hypoxia rescinded her level of consciousness improved. Her blood glucose levels were also recorded. They remained elevated around 9 mmol/l; however, this was regarded to be a stress response by the body, which would be self-limiting.

Exposure

Winnie was provided with mouthcare and eye care when she received oxygen therapy and NIPPV to prevent her mouth and eyes becoming dry and ulcerated. She was given comfort breaks from the NIPPV face mask at hourly intervals. Winnie was nursed on a low air-loss mattress and turned regularly to prevent pressure sores developing.

CASE STUDY 5.3: ASTHMA – BIJU JACOB

Case study 5.3 takes a look at a patient who has been admitted with an acute exacerbation of asthma. 5.4 million people in the UK are currently receiving treatment for asthma and on average three people a day die from asthma (Asthma UK, 2016).

Acute severe asthma is defined as the presence of more than one of the following symptoms: wheeze, breathlessness, chest tightness, cough, and of variable airflow obstruction (BTS, 2016). Airway hyper-responsiveness and airway inflammation are also now regarded to be key symptoms (BTS, 2016).

Activity 5.9

Read the following case study. What is asthma?

Biju had been treated for a mild chest infection by his GP. However, today he attended his doctors, having deteriorated. The GP diagnosed acute severe asthma (BTS, 2016) and he was admitted to a medical ward at the local hospital. A summary of his observations is presented in Box 5.9.

Box 5.9 Biju's initial assessment

Biju Jacob (57) is a known smoker and notoriously non-compliant with his asthma medication. He has been seen by his GP this morning who has been managing his asthma; however his condition has deteriorated over the past five days. Biju has been admitted to a medical ward with severe, acute asthma.

Airway

- Biju was just about able to speak in short sentences
- Peak expiratory flow rate is 200 (Biju's normal is 500)
- Trachea central
- Poor air entry bilaterally with widespread wheeze and crackles at the right base
- Chest resonant to percussion bilaterally with a small area of dullness at the right base
- There is no productive cough

Breathing

- Respiratory rate 30 breaths per minute (bpm) and accessory muscles are being used
- Oxygen saturation levels: 91% on air

Circulation

- Heart rate 120 bpm
- Blood pressure 120/75 mmHg
- Capillary refill 2 secs
- Biju is apyrexial
- Urine output was a cumulative 145 mls over the past three hours

Disability

- Biju is A on ACVPU but he looks frightened and scared
- There are no complaints of pain
- Blood sugar 6.7 mmol/l

Exposure

- Pressure areas intact
- Biju has one green peripheral line in situ

Acute severe asthma

Based on the BTS Guidelines (2017), acute severe asthma is diagnosed by any one of the following:

1. A peak expiratory flow (PEF) rate of 33–50%. A PEF is a measure of the maximum speed of expiration. Measured through a flow meter it measures the flow through the bronchi and provides an indication of the degree of obstruction in the airway. PEF is expressed as a % of the patient's previous recorded best value.
2. A respiratory rate equal to or greater than 25 breaths per minute.
3. A tachycardia of heart rate equal to or greater than 110 beats per minute.
4. An inability to complete sentences in one breath.

Activity 5.10

Describe the underlying pathophysiology.

Pathophysiology

Asthma causes bronchoconstriction which is the result of a sharp contraction of the smooth muscle in the airways which causes the trachea, the bronchi and the bronchioles to narrow. This is the result of damage to the layer of cells which line the airway – the airway epithelium. This damage can also contribute to the airways becoming hyper-responsive. This is because they lose their barrier function, which allows allergens to enter the airways and cause further inflammation. As the epithelium breaks down, sensory nerves become exposed, and they become stimulated. There is also a loss of enzymes that break down inflammatory mediators meaning the airways remain inflamed (Kaufman, 2011). Changes can also occur in the subepithelial layer, which loses its elasticity as collagen fibres build up. This causes the airways to become stiff and poorly compliant and highly resistant to airflow (Rees, 2010).

In asthma, there is also over-production of mucus, oedema, bronchospasm, and muscle damage (Kaufman, 2011). This is the result of asthma causing the airway's mucus-secreting cells to multiply and the mucous glands to enlarge. This results in increased mucus secretion which helps form mucous plugs that can block off the airways (Ward et al., 2015).

The capillaries in the airway walls can dilate and there can also be increased capillary permeability. This will result in oedema developing in the airways and an increase in airway secretions. There will also be an impaired clearance of mucous and the development of oedema, which may also contribute to narrowing of the airways and hyper-responsiveness (Kaufman, 2011).

With poorly controlled chronic asthma, changes in structural cells and tissues can occur in the lower respiratory tract. This results in permanent fibrotic damage which can lead to long-term damage to the airways involving a reduction in airway compliance and an increase in airway resistance (Rees, 2010).

MANAGEMENT OF AN ACUTE SEVERE EXACERBATION OF ASTHMA

Management of acute exacerbations of asthma in the UK is driven by a number of national drivers including:

- NICE NG *80 Asthma: Diagnosis, monitoring and chronic asthma management* (NICE, 2017b)
- NICE *Asthma Clinical Knowledge Summary* (CKS) (NICE, 2018).
- BTS/SIGN *British guideline on the management of asthma* (BTS/SIGN, 2019)

Activity 5.11

Discuss the management plan for Biju based upon the National Drivers and evidence base.

Assessment

Following on from the A–E assessment presented in Box 5.9, Biju was put on hourly observations using the National Early Warning Score (2) (RCP, 2017). This found Biju had a very high NEWS2 score of 9 which necessitated immediate referral to an emergency response team such as the critical care outreach team (RCP, 2017). This was because Biju was at great risk of rapid deterioration.

Airway

The priority was to treat Biju's airway obstruction as the team did not want this to deteriorate further. This was managed through the administration of nebulized 5 mg of salbutamol over 30–60 minutes.

The salbutamol was administered through a continuous pressurised oxygen-driven nebuliser unit (flow rate of 6 l /min usually needed) to prevent Biju's hypoxia worsening (BTS/SIGN, 2019).

Salbutamol is a short-acting Beta2 agonist that works on the Beta2 adrenergic receptors in the smooth muscle of bronchus and bronchioles. This results in bronchodilation and relieves chest tightness and breathlessness (Scullion & Holmes, 2010).

As Biju had severe acute asthma nebulised ipratropium bromide (0.5 mg 4–6 hourly) was also administered (BTS/SIGN, 2019). This is a bronchodilator, which provides an 'anti-cholinergic' effect by blocking the actions of acetyl choline (Ach) on the smooth muscle of the bronchi causing it to dilate.

Breathing

As Biju's airway was being managed with the nebulisers an arterial blood gas was taken. The results are presented in Box 5.10.

Box 5.10 Arterial blood gas result

pH 7.32

PaO_2 6.8 kPa

$PaCO_2$ 6.4 kPa

HCO_3 –28 mmol/l

Lactate 2 mmol/l

BE 2

SaO_2 91%

Activity 5.12

Analyse the arterial blood gas result. What does it show?

Once the nebulisers had finished, Biju was administered controlled supplementary oxygen via a fixed-performance oxygen mask (BTS/ SIGN, 2019), in this case a venturi mask. As Biju's ABG result identified hypoxaemia, Biju was commenced on 35% oxygen at 8 litres per minute via the venturi mask. The ABG was reassessed when his oxygen saturation level reached 94–98% (BTS/ SIGN, 2019). Biju was also commenced on a short course of steroid therapy. As he was able to swallow, he received a five-day course of 40–50 mg of oral prednisolone. If Biju had been unable to swallow, he would have received an intramuscular injection of methylprednisolone 160 mg or IV hydrocortisone 100 mg (NICE, 2018). These steroids reduce inflammation and decrease airway hyper-responsiveness (Holgate & Douglass, 2010). Because there were no signs of infection, Biju did not receive antibiotics (NICE, 2018).

Following administration of the bronchodilators, steroids and oxygen, Biju's ABGs after four hours were as shown in Box 5.11.

Box 5.11 Arterial blood gas result

pH 7.35

PaO_2 9.2 kPa

$PaCO_2$ 4.9 kPa

HCO_3 –28 mmol/l

Lactate 2 mmol/l

BE 2

SaO_2 94%

Activity 5.13

Analyse the next arterial blood gas result. What does it show?

Slowly, the amount of oxygen Biju received via the venturi mask was reduced to 28%. However, this was administered through a humidification system to prevent Biju's airways from drying out and further exacerbating any inflammation. His saturations continued to be monitored with the aim that they remained at 94% or above.

Circulation

Biju was tachycardiac on admission to the ward and not too keen on drinking. As his respiratory rate was 30 breaths per minute and with a NEWS2 of nine, he was commenced on IV fluids at a maintenance rate of 25–30 mls/kg/day (NICE, 2017b). This was calculated for him to be 2–2.4 litres per day. There was no pyrexia present, and his capillary refill time was within normal limits. Biju was able to mobilise to the toilet; however, he was commenced on a strict fluid balance chart and his fluid input and output was recorded with a cumulative balance calculated. The aim was for Biju to be in a slightly positive balance for the first 24 hours to make up for a fluid deficit that had been developing over the previous days. Ultimately the aim was for him to be in a neutral fluid balance.

Disability

As his condition improved, Biju became less anxious. His ACVPU remained good and he was able to interact with his family who had come to visit. His blood sugar levels were monitored six hourly and remained within normal limits.

Exposure

Initially, Biju was nursed at 30° to reduce the risk of aspiration. His skin was clean and intact; however, Biju was encouraged to turn himself in bed every two hours to reduce the risk of him developing pressure sores with a view to him mobilising gently as soon as his condition improved. His cannula site has a Visual Infusion Phlebitis (VIP) score of 0 and was observed daily throughout his admission.

The BTS/SIGN (2019) guidelines identify that patients with severe asthma and one or more adverse psychosocial factors are at risk of death. Consequently, prior to his discharge back to the care of his GP, Biju was referred to the smoking cessation clinic to provide him with the necessary psychosocial support to quit smoking.

SUMMARY

This chapter has presented three patient scenarios for patients experiencing difficulties with breathing. The chapter has explained how to use the ABCDE approach to prioritise care and to plan interventions based upon the evidence base. The following chapter will now proceed to explore circulation.

REFERENCES

Baraldo, S., Turato, G. & Saetta M. (2012) Pathophysiology of the small airways in chronic obstructive pulmonary disease. *Respiration*, 84, 89–97.

BMJ Best Practice (2020) *Community-acquired pneumonia (non COVID-19) – symptoms, diagnosis and treatment.* Available at: https://bestpractice.bmj.com/topics/en-gb/3000108 (accessed 24 January 2022).

BMJ Best Practice (2021) COPD. Available at: https://bestpractice.bmj.com/topics/en-gb/7 (accessed 24 January 2022).

BTS (2009) *BTS guidelines for the management of community acquired pneumonia in adults: Update 2009.* Available at: https://thorax.bmj.com/content/64/Suppl_3/iii1 (accessed 24 January 2022).

BTS (2016) BTS/ICS guidelines for the ventilatory management of acute hypercapnic respiratory failure in adults. *Thorax*, 71, ii1–ii35.

BTS (2017) *Oxygen therapy guidelines.* Available at: https://www.brit-thoracic.org.uk/quality-improvement/guidelines/emergency-oxygen/ (accessed 24 January 2022).

BTS/SIGN (2019) *British guideline on the management of asthma.* Available at: www.sign.ac.uk/media/1773/sign158-updated.pdf (accessed 24 January 2022).

Clancy, J. & McVicar, A. (2009) *Physiology and Anatomy for Nurses and Healthcare Practitioners: A Homeostatic Approach* (3rd ed.). London: Hodder Arnold.

Cutler, L. & Cutler, J. (2010) *Critical Care Nursing Made Incredibly Easy*. Riverwoods, IL: Lippincott Williams and Wilkin.

Gibson, V. (2015) Recognising and managing community-acquired pneumonia. *Nursing Standard*, 30 (12), 53–60.

Hill Bailey, P., McMillan Boyles, C., Duff Cloutier, J., Bartlett, A., Goodridge, D., Manji, M. & Dusek, B. (2013) *Nursing Care of Dyspnoea: The 6th Vital Sign in Individuals with Chronic Obstructive Pulmonary Disease (COPD)*. Ontario: Registered Nurses' Association of Ontario.

Holgate, S.T. & Douglass, J. (2010) *Fast Facts: Asthma* (3rd ed.). Oxford: Health Press Ltd.

Hooper, R., Burney, P., Vollmer, W. M., McBurnie, M. A., Gislason, T., Tan, W. C., Jithoo, A., Kocabas, A., Weltee, T. & Buist, A. S. (2012) Risk factors for COPD spirometrically defined from the lower limit of normal in the BOLD project. *European Journal of Respiration*, 39, 1343–1353.

Kaufman, G. (2011) Asthma: pathophysiology, diagnosis and management. *Nursing Standard*. 26 (5) 48–56

Mitchell, J. (2015) Pathophysiology of COPD: Part 2. *Practice Nursing*, 26 (9), 444–449.

Morgan, A.J. & Glossop, A.J. (2016) Severe community-acquired pneumonia. *BJA Education*, 16 (5), 167–172.

NCEPOD (2015) *Just say sepsis*. Available at: www.ncepod.org.uk/2015report2/downloads/JustSaySepsis_FullReport.pdf (accessed 24 January 2022).

NHS Digital (2018) *Health survey for England*. Available at: https://digital.nhs.uk/data-and-information/publications/statistical/health-survey-for-england/2018 (accessed 24 January 2022).

NHS England (2012) *An outcomes strategy for COPD and Asthma: NHS companion document*. Available at: https://assets.publishing.service.gov.uk/government/uploads/system/uploads/attachment_data/file/216531/dh_134001.pdf (accessed 24 January 2022).

NHS England (2018) *Chronic Obstructive Pulmonary Disease (COPD) pathway*. Available at: www.england.nhs.uk/rightcare/products/pathways/chronic-obstructive-pulmonary-disease-copd-pathway/ (accessed 24 January 2022).

NICE (2014) *Pneumonia in adults*. Available at: www.nice.org.uk/guidance/qs110/chapter/quality-statement-1-mortality-risk-assessment-in-primary-care-using-crb65-score (accessed 24 January 2022).

NICE (2017a) *Sepsis: Recognition, diagnosis and early management NG 51*. Available at: www.nice.org.uk/guidance/NG51 (accessed 24 January 2022).

NICE (2017b) *Asthma: diagnosis, monitoring and chronic asthma management NG 80*. Available at: www.nice.org.uk/guidance/ng80 (accessed 24 January 2022).

NICE (2018) Chronic Obstructive Pulmonary Disease in the over 16s: diagnosis and management. NG115. Available at: https://www.nice.org.uk/guidance/ng115 (accessed 23 February 2022).

Peate, I. & Dutton, H. (2021) *Acute Nursing Care: Recognising and Responding to Medical Emergencies* (2nd ed.). London: Routledge.

Rees, J. (2010) Asthma control in adults. In J. Rees, D. Kanabar & S. Pattini (Eds.), *ABC of Asthma* (6th ed.) (pp. 1–54). Chichester: John Wiley and Sons.

RCP (2017) *National Early Warning Score 2*. Available at: www.rcplondon.ac.uk/projects/outputs/national-early-warning-score-news-2 (accessed 24 January 2022).

Scullion, J. & Holmes, S. (2010) Prescribing beta-agonists for respiratory disease. *Independent Nurse*, 19 April, 22–24.

Sepsis Trust (2019) *Sepsis Six*. Available at: https://sepsistrust.org/about/about-sepsis/ (accessed 24 January 2022).

Ward, J. P. T., Ward, J. & Leach, R. M. (2015) *The Respiratory System at a Glance* (4th ed.). Chichester: Blackwell.

6

CIRCULATION – ANATOMY, PHYSIOLOGY AND PATHOPHYSIOLOGY

ALICE SKULL

Chapter learning outcomes

By the end of this chapter you will be able to:

1. Identify the main functions of the cardiovascular system.
2. Understand the homeostatic regulation of the body: cardiac output, stroke volume, mean arterial pressure and systemic vascular resistance.
3. Examine fluid physiology and the relationship to maintain homeostasis.
4. Understand how the body regulates temperature.
5. Explain the function of the innate and adaptive immune system.
6. Analyse the concept 'Acute coronary syndrome' and discuss the underpinning pathophysiology.
7. Describe the underlying physiological mechanisms that occur with each type of shock.
8. Explore the underlying pathophysiology relating to sepsis.
9. Discuss the pathophysiology of Acute Kidney Injury.

Key words

- Systole
- Diastole
- Preload

(Continued)

- Cardiac output
- Stroke volume
- Renin Angiotensin Aldosterone mechanism
- Conduction system
- Fluid balance
- Vasoconstriction
- Vasodilation
- White blood cells
- Coronary arteries
- Hypovolaemic shock
- Cardiogenic shock
- Obstructive shock
- Distributive shock
- Anaphylactic
- Septic
- Neurogenic
- Acute kidney injury

INTRODUCTION

The cardiovascular system is often referred to as the transport system for the body comprising of a pump (the heart), the pipes (blood vessels) and the fluid (blood). This chapter will consider the role of the cardiovascular system in supplying the body with the necessary oxygen, fluid and nutrient requirements, focusing on the systemic and pulmonary circulation, the cardiac cycle and electrical innervation of the heart. Regulation of fluid balance, thermoregulation and the immune system will be considered before an introduction to acute coronary system pathophysiology, shock, acute kidney injury, sepsis and anaphylaxis are introduced. The following chapter will develop this understanding of pathophysiology with application to patient scenarios.

The heart is a truly amazing organ, pumping ceaselessly through the day yet we are largely unaware of its action. It is an incredibly effective small muscular pump, the size of a fist. The heart is actually two pumps, side by side (Figure 6.1). The right side of the heart receives deoxygenated blood from the body tissues via the superior and inferior vena cava and coronary sinus and then pumps this blood to the lungs to pick up oxygen and to dispel carbon dioxide. The blood vessels carrying blood to and from the lungs form the pulmonary circuit. The left side of the heart receives oxygenated blood returning from the lungs and pumps this blood via the aorta to the body, supplying each cell with oxygen and nutrients for life. The blood vessels that carry blood to and from the body form the systemic circuit. Blood vessels, unlike the pipes of a household plumbing system are not rigid tubes but are capable of bending, flexing, constricting and relaxing.

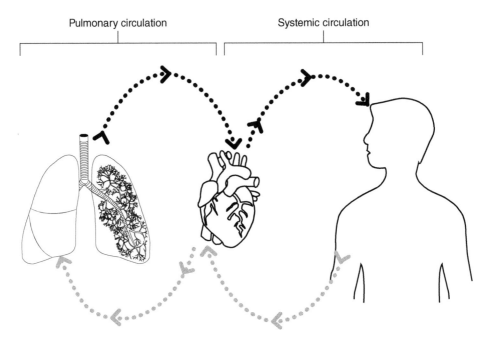

Figure 6.1 Systemic and pulmonary circuit

The three major types of blood vessels are arteries, capillaries and veins. Arteries carry blood away from the heart and veins carry blood towards the heart. In the systemic circulation, arteries always carry oxygenated blood and veins carry deoxygenated blood. The opposite is true in the pulmonary circuit.

These vessels within the circulatory system provide the body with the network by which nutrients and oxygen and waste/toxins are transported. Blood is pumped from the heart into the major arteries of the body. These branch to form increasingly smaller arteries and eventually arterioles. The latter are continuous with a close-mesh network of vessels, the capillaries which have direct contact with the tissue cells. Blood then passes into larger vessels, which join with one another to form veins; these unite to form the largest veins, which take the blood back into the heart.

ARTERIES

Arteries vary in minute structure according to their size, location and role, but all possess three layers/coverings: the tunica intima (inner), tunica media (middle) and tunica adventitia (outer).

- The tunica intima contains the endothelium that lines the lumen of all vessels. Its flat surface minimizes friction as the blood moves through the lumen. It is a key protective lining of the vessel.
- The tunica media consists of a series of circular elastic membranes, separated by fibrous tissue that encloses smooth muscle cells. It is the bulkiest of the three layers but its activities are critical in regulating circulatory dynamics because small changes in vessel diameter greatly influence blood flow and blood pressure.
- The tunica adventitia is composed of fibrous tissue containing a few elastic fibres that protect and reinforce the vessel, anchoring it to its surroundings.

In a person at rest, the heart pumps approximately 5 litres of blood into the vascular system every minute (discussed shortly). This cardiac output can increase to 30 litres/minute during strenuous exercise. The blood vessels must therefore be capable of accommodating large changes in cardiac output without sustaining any damage. It is for this reason that the arteries require thick, elastic walls. Marieb and Hoehn (2019) say they can be visualized as simple elastic tubes.

VEINS

The walls of the veins are composed of the same three layers as those of the arteries. However, the tunica media contains far fewer elastic and muscle fibres, resulting in a relatively inelastic structure. Their walls are always thinner as blood pressure within is lower, and their lumens larger than corresponding arteries. Most veins possess valves that prevent the reflux of blood. Each valve is pocket-like and formed from the tunica intima, covered by endothelium on both surfaces and strengthened by a connective tissue matrix.

Valves are usually paired and if regurgitation should occur the valves will become distended and the opposed edges brought into contact. The valves therefore effectively maintain a one-way blood flow within the venous system.

ARTERIOLES, VENULES AND CAPILLARIES

Blood flows from the arteries into arterioles, which represent the smallest of the arterial vessels. The tunica intima and media are thin while the adventitia increases in relative thickness.

Smaller arterioles that lead into capillary beds are little more than a single layer of smooth muscle cells spiralling around the endothelial lining (Marieb & Hoehn, 2019). Capillaries are the smallest blood vessels with exceedingly thin walls consisting just of a thin tunica intima. Average capillary length is 1 mm and average lumen diameter is 8–10 μm (Marieb & Hoehn, 2019). Blood passes from the capillary network into the venules, the smallest part of the venous system.

The capillaries are an extremely important part of the vascular system, since it is here that gaseous, nutritive and waste substances are exchanged with the tissues. Capillaries do not function independently – they form interweaving networks called capillary beds. The flow of blood from an arteriole to a venule is called 'microcirculation'. A metarteriole containing muscle fibres leads into a thoroughfare channel. This channel leads directly from arteriole to venule, and true capillaries open from them. The true capillaries are opened or closed by means of a precapillary sphincter (a valve regulating blood flow). If the sphincters are open, then blood flows through the true capillaries; when they are closed, blood flows through the metarteriole and thoroughfare. The precapillary sphincters are controlled by chemical substances locally in the tissues, unlike arterioles, which are innervated by the nervous system. A capillary bed may be flooded with blood or completely bypassed depending on the conditions in the body. For example, during vigorous exercise, blood is rerouted from your digestive system to the capillary beds of your skeletal muscles where it is more immediately needed.

The term *systole* refers to the contraction phase of the cardiac cycle and *diastole* refers to the relaxation phase. It is important to have an understanding of how the mechanical events of contraction and relaxation relate to the electrical innervation of the heart and movement of blood. Refer to the diagram of events during the cardiac cycle as you read the following section. The *cardiac cycle* includes all events associated with blood flow through the heart during one complete heartbeat. During mid to late diastole, the ventricles are filling with blood and the heart is in total relaxation. Blood returns from the circulation passively through the atria and open atrioventricular valves into the ventricles. The pulmonary and aortic valves are closed; more than 80% of ventricular filling occurs during this period (Marieb & Hoehn, 2019). The remaining 20% is delivered when the atria contract. This ventricular volume after filling is referred to as *End Diastolic Volume (EDV)* and is helpful in understanding later discussion of the clinical term *preload*. Depolarisation of the atria gives rise to the 'p wave' on the ECG. As the atria relax, the ventricles begin contracting. There is a sharp rise in ventricular pressure as the atrioventricular valves close and the ventricles are now completely closed chambers for a split second. Depolarisation of the ventricles gives rise to the QRS waveform on the ECG. Systemic vascular resistance has to be overcome to force open the pulmonary and aortic valves. Blood flow is initially very rapid with aorta pressure normally reaching about 120 mmHg; as contraction wanes, ejection is reduced. Ventricular repolarisation gives rise to the T wave on the ECG. In early diastole the ventricles relax and blood in the aorta starts to backflow into the left ventricle. The heart is never entirely empty; the volume of blood remaining in the ventricles is referred to as *End Systolic Volume (ESV)*. Closure of the aortic semi-lunar valve causes a brief rise in aortic pressure as back-flowing blood rebounds off the valve cusps seen as a dicrotic notch on the pressure graph. The ventricles are now totally closed. When atrial blood pressure on the atrial side of the atrioventricular valves exceeds that in the ventricles, the atrioventricular valves are forced open and ventricular filling begins once again.

Activity 6.1

Print out a rhythm strip from a cardiac monitor of a patient you have looked after. Can you identify the PQRST waves?

Cardiac output is the amount of blood pumped out by each ventricle in 1 minute. It is the product of heart rate and stroke volume. *Stroke volume* is the volume of blood pumped out by one ventricle with each beat. As the left ventricle is the dominant force in the heart, it is usually used to calculate stroke volume and cardiac output. Using normal resting values for the heart, the average adult cardiac output can be calculated as in Figure 6.2.

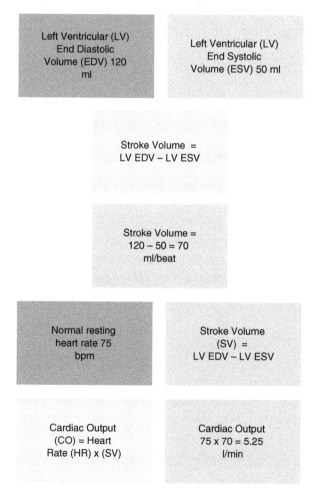

Figure 6.2   Average adult cardiac output calculation

The normal adult blood volume is about 5 litres (Marieb & Hoehn, 2019). Therefore, we can see that the entire blood supply passes through each side of the heart once each minute.

This correlation between heart rate and stroke volume is important to appreciate as cardiac output varies directly with stroke volume and heart rate. When stroke volume increases or the heart beats faster or both, cardiac output increases and conversely when either factor decreases. Major factors enhance cardiac output, for example, exercise stimulates activity of the respiratory pump, skeletal muscle activity and causes increased sympathetic venous constriction, which in turn speeds venous return. Stroke volume is controlled by the degree of stretch of the heart muscle, referred to as *preload*. The relationship between preload and stroke volume is called the *Frank-Starling law of the heart*, often referred to as the law of elasticity. The greater the degree of stretch of cardiac muscle, the greater the force of contraction. The key determinant of stretch of heart muscle is venous return, the amount of blood returning to the heart. *Contractility* is a further key determinant of cardiac output and is governed by chemical change, namely calcium uptake from the sarcoplasmic reticulum and chemical stimulation from positive inotropic agents such as adrenaline, thyroxine, glucagon and the drug digoxin.

Activity 6.2

Using the BNF, review the action of adrenaline, thyroxine, glucagon and digoxin.

A key measure of cardiac function and effectiveness is measurement of blood pressure. Blood pressure describes the force exerted on a vessel wall and is expressed in mmHg. The peak pressure generated during the contraction phase of the heart is called the *systolic pressure* and the lowest pressure is referred to as *diastolic pressure*. The difference between the systolic and diastolic pressures is called the *pulse pressure*. Arterial blood pressure reflects two factors:

- How much the elastic arteries close to the heart can stretch.
- The volume of blood forced into them (Marieb & Hoehn, 2019).

We have seen that aortic pressures fluctuate with each heartbeat, so an important indicator of pressure is the *Mean Arterial Pressure (MAP)*. As diastole usually lasts longer than systole, MAP is roughly equal to the diastolic pressure plus one-third of the pulse pressure:

$$\text{MAP} = \text{diastolic pressure} + \frac{\text{pulse pressure}}{3}$$

For a person with a systolic blood pressure of 120 mmHg and a diastolic pressure of 80 mmHg:

$$\text{MAP} = 80 \text{ mmHg} + \frac{40 \text{ mmHg}}{3} = 93 \text{ mmHg}$$

The body continually manipulates this equation to maintain adequate perfusion and achieve homeostasis. The main factors determining cardiac output are venous return (EDV) and the neural and hormonal controls. The cardiac centre in the medulla is in charge of heart rate, via the parasympathetic vagus nerves; during rest (as opposed to exercise/stress), venous return largely controls stroke volume. During exercise or stress the cardioacceleratory centre takes over, activating the sympathetic nervous system, increasing heart rate by acting on the sinoatrial (SA) node, releasing adrenaline and increasing stroke volume by enhancing contractility, which decreases EDV. Increased heart rate and increased stroke volume enhance cardiac output (CO = SV x HR), in turn increasing MAP. This continual adjustment maintains a MAP of 65 mmHg+ to maintain end organ perfusion. Long term regulation of blood pressure occurs via the kidneys.

Key neural control of blood pressure involves the action of stretch receptors called *baro-receptors*. The prefix 'baro' refers to pressure like a barometer that may be found in the home to measure atmospheric pressure as an indicator of change in the weather. Baroreceptors are located in areas of significant blood flow, in the carotid sinuses and aortic arch. Baroreceptors detect change in blood pressure and when stretched send a barrage of messages to the medulla, inducing vasodilation. When blood pressure falls, baroreceptor activity is inhibited and cardioacceleratory functions are stimulated causing vasoconstriction and an increase in resistance. Located in the same areas are *chemoreceptors*, which detect chemical changes, such as changes in pH, oxygen saturation and carbon dioxide levels. Chemoreceptors play a larger role in regulating respiratory rate than blood pressure and are considered within the breathing physiology chapter.

The kidneys also have a key role in the regulation of blood pressure and understanding of the *renin–angiotensin–aldosterone mechanism* is key to understanding this and the compensatory mechanisms that occur in acute illness. Unlike short-term controls of blood pressure that alter peripheral resistance and cardiac output, long term controls alter blood volume (Marieb & Hoehn, 2019). The direct renal mechanism alters blood volume independently of hormones. When blood pressure or blood volume rises, the rate of glomerular filtration increases and filtrate cannot be reabsorbed rapidly enough, resulting in an increase in urine formation. In contrast, when blood pressure is low, water is conserved, reabsorbed and blood pressure rises. The kidneys can also regulate blood pressure indirectly via the renin–angiotensin–aldosterone mechanism (see Figure 6.3).

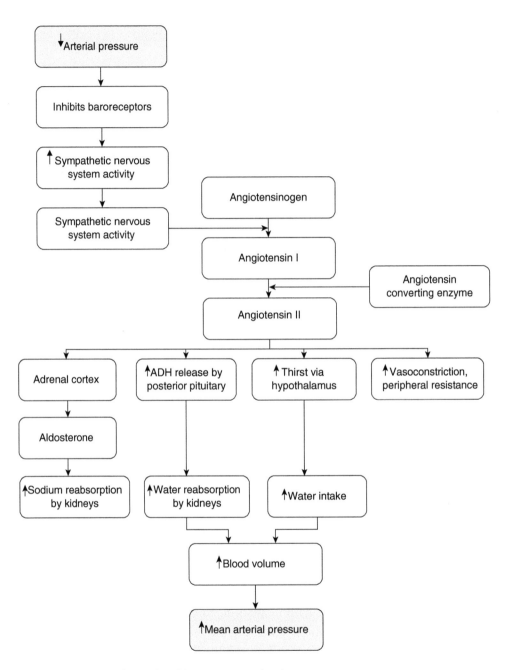

Figure 6.3   Renin–angiotensin–aldosterone mechanism

When arterial pressure falls, juxtaglomerular cells in the kidney release the enzyme renin. Renin interacts with angiotensinogen, a plasma protein made in the liver converting it into angiotensin I. Angiotensin converting enzyme (ACE) converts angiotensin I into angiotensin II. *Remember ACE –* it is key to the understanding of the first line anti-hypertensive drug group ACE Inhibitors (NICE, 2019a). Angiotensin II has four key effects on regulation of blood pressure and fluid volume. It stimulates the adrenal cortex to secrete aldosterone, an anti-natriuretic, which increases sodium reabsorption by the kidneys. Where sodium goes, water follows and therefore blood volume and blood pressure increase. Angiotensin II also causes the posterior pituitary gland to release anti-diuretic hormone, resulting in more water reabsorption. *Note this – this anti-diuretic hormone* is also called *Vasopressin*, a pharmacological agent used in clinical practice. Look up the term diabetes insipidus and how this relates to the anti-diuretic hormone.

The third action of angiotensin II is the activation of the thirst mechanism in the hypo-thalamus. Lastly and importantly, angiotensin II is a potent vasoconstrictor, increasing blood pressure by increasing peripheral resistance.

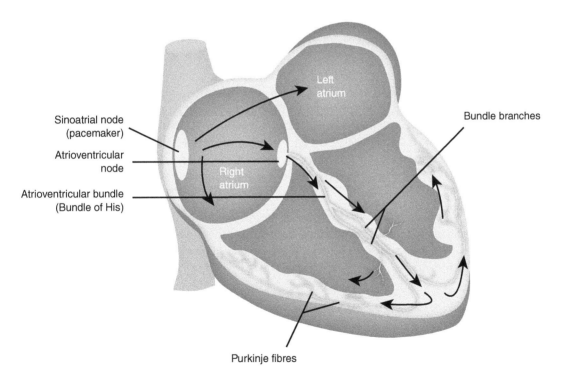

Figure 6.4 Electrical conduction system

The heart works under electrical innervation, giving rise to the mechanical events of blood through the heart discussed above. Specialised electrical fibres have the intrinsic ability to generate electrical activity and pass it on to make the heart muscle contract. ECG tracings arise from the electrical changes that accompany muscle contraction. With knowledge of the normal anatomy and physiology of the heart, its conduction systems and the relative position of the leads to the electrodes, you will improve your monitoring skills and understanding.

The heart is typically described as a 'blunt inverted cone', the size of the owner's fist. This means that impulses, triggered from the Sino Atrial (SA) node, travel from the base down to the apex. The impulses travel back up the ventricular walls via the Purkinje fibres, causing the heart to depolarise towards the valves at the top of the chamber – so maximising output (if depolarisation only occurred from the base, the contraction wave would squeeze the blood in the wrong direction – which can occur with ectopic activity).

The left ventricle is larger in volume and muscle mass than the right ventricle, therefore the conductive system is more extensive, with the Left Bundle Branch being divided into two fascicles to ensure the heart contracts as one functional syncytium. Impulses can thus be spread more quickly through the muscle mass.

The *Sinoatrial (SA) node* is a specialized collection of cells situated near the junction of the superior vena cava with the right atrium and is responsible for setting the pace of the heart rhythm. Note – it is helpful to remember that the SA node is often referred to as the heart's natural pacemaker as it is a reminder that the treatment for rhythm disturbance in the heart can sometimes be a surgically inserted pacemaker. It receives its instructions from the sympathetic (adrenaline response) and parasympathetic (vagus nerve) systems depending on the demands placed on the heart by the needs of the body. It generates approximately 75 beats per minute (bpm).

From the SA node the depolarization spreads across the atria via the intermodal pathways to the *Atrioventricular (AV) node*. The AV node is a collection of cells, which lies at the junction of the right atrium with the ventricular septum. The impulse is delayed for 0.10s, allowing time for the atria to fill the ventricles. Its intrinsic discharge rate is slower than the SA node at approximately 60 bpm.

The *Bundle of His* (atrioventricular bundle) is the continuity of the AV node through the fibrous ring separating the atria and the ventricles. It is the only electrical connection between the atria and the ventricles. The electrical wave sweeping through the Bundle of His allows for ventricular filling to be completed by the atria.

The *right and left bundle branches* travel down the interventricular septum toward the heart apex, supplying electrical activity to the ventricles. The anterior fascicle of the left bundle branch supplies the anterior and superior left ventricle, whilst the posterior fascicle supplies the inferior and posterior left ventricle. The wave of depolarization spreads from left to right across the septum.

The *Purkinje fibres* or the terminating fibres of the conduction system enclose the whole of the ventricular muscle, creating a closed network of conduction and ensure the wave of electrical conduction reaches the outermost aspects of the cardiac muscle.

This pathway of electrical conduction can be viewed as the motorway route of conduction – the most effective and efficient way to make the heart contract. In contrast, in episodes of arrhythmia, the conduction pathway can be viewed as 'taking the country lanes' – sometimes this results in a 'short cut' and the rhythm seen is a tachycardia; at other times the country lanes take a longer route and the rhythm seen is a bradycardia.

Understanding of the 'motorway' electrical pathway can now be applied to the view that is seen on an ECG (Figure 6.5).

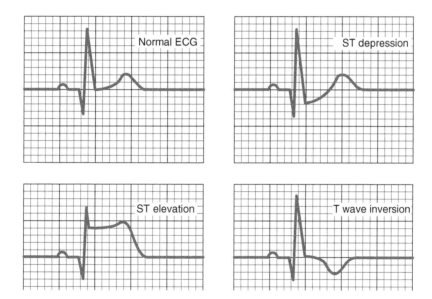

Figure 6.5   PQRST wave

The small p wave represents depolarisation of the atria, initiated by the SA node. A normal p wave is rounded and upright in appearance reflecting its origin in the SA node. The much larger QRS complex reflects the depolarisation of the ventricles. The normal duration of the QRS complex is <0.12s. The T wave represents ventricular repolarisation (repolarisation of the atria is masked by the QRS complex). Repolarisation is slower than depolarisation so the T wave is more spread out and smaller than the QRS complex. Further measurement that may be of significance in rhythm interpretation clinically is measurement of the PR interval, which should be between 0.12s and 0.2s, and the QT interval, which should be between 0.35s and 0.45s.

Activity 6.3

Select a 12-lead ECG from practice or use a text book example to apply this description of the PQRST waves.

FLUID PHYSIOLOGY

Principles of fluid physiology are based on a balance between fluid loss and fluid gain.

- Gastro-intestinal tract – represents both gain through drinking and water from food and also loss through excretion of faecal matter.
- Skin – represents insensible loss through sweating and processes of metabolic activity.
- Renal – sees loss through excretion of urine.
- Respiratory – loss through expiration.

Average water intake and output should be in homeostatic balance. Water within the body contains electrolytes, which are substances that develop an electrical charge when dissolved in water. There are two categories of electrolyte:

- Cation – positive ions such as Na+, Ca+ and K+.
- Anion – negative ions such as CL-, HCO_3^-.

These ions have a role in the regulation of fluid balance and acid base balance essential to neuromuscular excitability, neuronal function and enzyme reaction. Therefore fluid balance is key for these functions to be maintained. The concentration of these solutes in the body is called *osmolarity*.

Fluid represents 60% of body weight in the average man and 50% in the average female. There are two major fluid compartments of the body – intracellular fluid (ICF), which makes up 40% of the body weight, and extracellular fluid (ECF), which makes up 20% of body weight. Extracellular fluid can be further divided into interstitial fluid (80% of ECF) and plasma (20% of ECF). Regulation of fluid balance ensures that the body's water is present and distributed proportionally among all the compartments (picture measuring scales). When more water is lost than is gained from the body, this is referred to as *dehydration*. Dehydration results when 1% or more of body weight is lost through fluid loss. This means there is not enough fluid in the interstitial compartments and results in an increase in osmolarity and the thirst centre in the hypothalamus is stimulated. Stimulation of the thirst centre is another good example of the body's ability to be able to compensate for loss and preserve body function. Osmoreceptors in the hypothalamus are stimulated causing an increase in thirst and water uptake and dehydration is then relieved. People of all ages can become severely dehydrated through diarrhoea and vomiting and this tends to be considered as a developing world problem – however is also responsible for a significant number of deaths in the developed world (WHO, 2018), contributing to fluid imbalance and acute kidney injury.

Regulation of fluid balance is achieved through three principle mechanisms:

- Renal regulation – renin-angiotensin-aldosterone mechanism
- Cardiac control
- Pituitary control

Stimulation of the renin-angiotensin-aldosterone mechanism has been previously discussed in relation to regulation of blood pressure and the same mechanism is also stimulated in response to decreased tissue perfusion.

When blood volume and blood pressure rise and begin to stretch the atria as fluid returns to the heart, Atrial Natriuretic Peptide (ANP) that is stored in the atria shuts off the renin-angiotensin-aldosterone system, which stabilizes blood and blood pressure. ANP thereby acts as the counterbalance to the renin-angiotensin-aldosterone mechanism.

We also noted earlier the effect of the anti-diuretic hormone released from the pituitary gland on reabsorption of water – another factor in the regulation of fluid balance.

Osmotic and hydrostatic pressures regulate the continuous exchange and mixing of body fluids (Marieb & Hoehn, 2019). Think of this as 'push' and 'pull'.

- **Hydrostatic pressure** is the force exerted by fluid pushing against a blood vessel wall. Think of it like the weight of water pushing against the wall of a dam in a river. In capillaries, hydrostatic pressure forces fluid through the capillary walls – this is called *filtration*.
- **Colloid osmotic pressure** is the force opposing hydrostatic pressure. It is created by large molecules such as proteins that are unable to cross the capillary walls. These proteins, like Albumin, have a magnetic effect to water and pull water towards them via *osmosis*.

Fluid filters from the capillaries at their arteriolar end and flows through the interstitial space. Most is *reabsorbed* at the venous end. A concentration gradient needs to exist between the blood and the tissue cells in order for the movement of solutes (*diffusion*) and the movement of water (osmosis) across the semi-permeable membrane to occur.

We thought about the mechanisms that correct dehydration, however the body is also subject to fluid volume excess. This is always the result of sodium and thus water gain. Hydrostatic pressure builds in the vessels and pushes water out. *Oedema* is the excessive accumulation of interstitial fluid. This can occur due to leakage at the vessel site due to puncturing the skin, increased capillary permeability, decreased concentration of plasma proteins resulting in a low colloid osmotic pressure, damage to the cell membrane or an increase in extracellular fluid. We will consider this increased capillary permeability and resulting fluid shift when we consider sepsis pathophysiology.

THERMOREGULATION

With the current focus on identification and management of sepsis it is very important to underpin this understanding with an awareness of how the body regulates temperature and also then go on to consider the immune system.

Body temperature is another homeostatic mechanism, representing the balance between heat production and heat loss. All body tissues produce heat with the most metabolically active producing the greatest amounts. At rest, most heat is generated by the:

- Liver
- Heart
- Brain
- Kidneys
- Endocrine organs (Marieb & Hoehn, 2019)

The inactive skeletal muscles account for only 20–30%. Slight changes in muscle tone such as shivering change this dramatically and during vigorous exercise skeletal muscles can produce 30 to 40 times more heat than the rest of the body (Marieb & Hoehn, 2019). A change in muscle activity is one of the most important means of modifying body temperature.

Body temperature averages 37°C + 0.5°C and is usually maintained within the range 35.8°C–38.2°C (Marieb & Hoehn, 2019). A healthy individual's body temperature fluctuates approximately 1°C in 24 hours and is lowest in the early morning and highest in late afternoon or early evening. (Note – think about the time of day you have most frequently recorded a high temperature on a patient.) Each 1°C rise in temperature increases the rate of biochemical reactions by about 10% (Tortora & Derrickson, 2017).

Core temperature refers to body structures below the skin such as within the thorax and abdomen and is usually a little higher than the *shell temperature* (skin). In clinical nursing practice we are more likely to refer to 'shell temperature' as peripheral temperature. Core temperature is precisely regulated. Blood serves as the major agent of heat exchange between the core and the shell (Marieb & Hoehn, 2019). When the skin is warmer than the external environment, the body loses heat as blood flushes to the skin capillaries. Conversely, when heat must be conversed, blood largely bypasses the skin.

Heat always flows down a concentration gradient from a warmer region to a cooler region. The body uses four mechanisms of heat transfer:

- **Radiation** – the loss of heat in the form of infrared waves (thermal energy). Any object warmer than its environment will transfer heat to those objects. Close to half of body heat loss occurs by radiation (Marieb & Hoehn, 2019).
- **Conduction** – transfer heat from a warmer object to a cooler one.
- **Convection** – when cool air makes contact with the body, it becomes warmed and therefore less dense and is carried away. (Warm air expands and rises and cool air, being denser, falls.)
- **Evaporation** – the conversion of a liquid to a vapour. The evaporation of water from body surfaces removes large amounts of body heat. We identified earlier that some water loss is insensible (e.g. from the process of respiration from the lungs and oral mucosa); the accompanying heat loss is *insensible heat loss*. Evaporative heat loss becomes a *sensible* process when body temperature rises and sweating produces increased amounts of water for vaporisation.

The hypothalamus acts as a thermostat for the regulation of body temperature. It receives input from the *peripheral thermoreceptors* located in the skin and the *central thermoreceptors* sensitive to blood temperature, and is located in the body's core.

Heat promoting mechanisms instigated by the heat promoting centre in the hypothalamus are:

1. **Vasoconstriction** – diverting blood from skin capillaries to deeper tissues, minimising heat loss from skin surface.
2. **Shivering** – skeletal muscles activated to produce heat.
3. **Increase of metabolic rate** – sympathetic nervous system release of adrenaline and noradrenaline increase the metabolic rate and enhance heat production.

Heat loss mechanisms inhibiting the heat promoting centre in the hypothalamus and activating the heat loss centre are:

1. **Vasodilation** – as the blood vessels swell with warm blood, the skin loses heat by radiation, convection and conduction.
2. **Enhanced sweating** – sympathetic nervous system activates sweat glands to produce perspiration. As the water of the perspiration evaporates from the surface of the skin, the skin is cooled.

However, over exposure to a hot environment makes normal heat loss processes ineffective. The resulting *hyperthermia* (clinical term *pyrexia*), depresses the hypothalamus. At a core temperature of around 41°C, heat controlling mechanisms are suspended (Marieb & Hoehn, 2019). Increasing temperatures increase the metabolic rate, which increases heat production and multiple organ damage becomes a distinct possibility.

Fever is controlled hyperthermia (Marieb & Hoehn, 2019), triggered by the release of cytokines from damaged cells. Cell damage may be caused by infection, trauma, allergic reactions, cancer or CNS injuries. Cytokines cause the release of prostaglandins, which reset the hypothalamic thermostat to a higher than normal temperature so that heat promoting processes are initiated. Vasoconstriction prevents heat loss from the body's surface, the skin cools and shivering generates heat. The cold or chill stage of a fever is a sign that the body temperature will continue to rise until it reaches a new setting. It remains at the new setting until natural body defences or antibiotics reverse the disease process (Marieb & Hoehn, 2019).

Hypothermia is a low body temperature resulting from prolonged uncontrolled exposure to cold. As deterioration in temperature occurs, this is reflected in a slowing down of key body processes measured by recording vital signs (respiratory rate, blood pressure and heart rate). The individual becomes drowsy; shivering stops at a core temperature of 30–32°C when the body has exhausted its heat generating capabilities (Marieb & Hoehn, 2019). Uncorrected, hypothermia progresses to coma and ultimately death by cardiac arrest. (Note – conversely, therapeutic hypothermia following cardiac arrest is now recommended in resuscitation guidelines (Nolan et al., 2015) and supported by evidence-based research – see Arrich et al's (2016) systematic review of hypothermia for neuroprotection in adults after cardiopulmonary resuscitation, which found a favourable neurological outcome in the intervention group and a 30% survival benefit.)

IMMUNE SYSTEM

Immunity and the immune response can be best considered in terms of attack from an invader and defence by the body. Anatomy and physiology texts rely heavily on these military analogies to explain the immune response. The body has two intrinsic defensive systems that act both independently and cooperatively to provide resistance to disease or immunity:

1. The *innate (nonspecific) defence system* – the first line of defence is the skin and mucous membranes.
2. The second line of defence, when the first line has been penetrated, are *internal defences* such as antimicrobial proteins, phagocytes and other cells inhibiting invasion throughout the body, characterised by inflammation (Marieb & Hoehn, 2019).

The *adaptive (specific) defence system* – the third line of defence – takes longer to mobilise and targets specific foreign substances.

The skin is a formidable barrier to invading pathogens as are the mucous membranes that line all body cavities that open to the exterior (for example, the respiratory and urinary tract). In addition to this physical barrier, the skin and mucous membranes produce a variety of protective chemicals:

*   **Acid** – inhibit bacterial growth
*   **Enzymes** – found in saliva, respiratory mucus and lacrimal fluid of the eye (tears), destroy bacteria

- **Mucin** – sticky mucus traps many microbes
- **Defensins** – a broad-spectrum antimicrobial peptide secreted by skin and mucous membranes
- **Other chemicals** – such as sweat, which has a high concentration of fat and salt and is inhospitable to bacteria

The mucous membrane of the nose has mucus-coated hairs that trap invading particles and filter the air. *Cilia* in the upper respiratory tract propel inhaled dust and bacteria laden mucus towards the throat, preventing it from entering the lower respiratory tract.

Although this first line of defence is quite effective, it can be easily breached, and when this happens micro-organisms invade deeper tissues and the second line of defence comes into play.

Nonspecific internal defence mechanisms include phagocytes, natural killer cells, the inflammatory response, antimicrobial proteins and fever.

Pathogens that get through the skin or mucosae are confronted by *phagocytes. Neutrophils,* the most abundant type of white blood cell, become phagocytic ('phago' means to eat) on encountering infectious material in the tissues (Marieb & Hoehn, 2019). However, *macrophages* are the 'big eaters' of pathogens. They can be both freely circulating in the tissue spaces or stationary and permanently attached to a particular organ.

Natural killer cells are a unique group of defensive white blood cells that can lyse and kill cancer cells and virus-infected body cells before the adaptive defence mechanism kicks in. The name 'natural' killer cells reflect their nonspecificity compared to lymphocytes of the adaptive mechanism that target specific virus-infected or tumour cells (Marieb & Hoehn, 2019). Natural killer cells are not phagocytic – they kill the cell by programming it to die whilst also secreting potent chemicals that enhance the inflammatory response.

The inflammatory response is triggered in response to physical injury, chemicals, infection by viruses, fungi or bacteria or intense heat. It is a defensive mechanism usually characterised by four symptoms:

- Redness
- Heat
- Swelling
- Pain

A fifth symptom can be loss of function in the affected area.

The inflammatory response brings together a series of actions that explain these symptoms. Inflammatory chemicals are released by injured tissue cells into the interstitial fluid. An example of these would be mast cells releasing histamine. These inflammatory chemicals, including *kinins, prostaglandins* and *complement,* dilate local arterioles and create gaps in capillary walls, making them leaky.

Redness and heat are due to **vasodilation**, where the vessels become larger and congested with blood. Increased *permeability* also means that *exudate* seeps from the blood into the tissue spaces – a process called *extravasation* – and causes swelling, contributing to a sensation of pain due to pressure on nerve endings. This exudate brings much needed clotting factors, antibodies and proteins to the injury site.

Soon after inflammation begins, phagocytes flood the injury area with neutrophils taking the lead, followed by macrophages. Neutrophils stick to the surface of the endothelium of blood vessels – a process called *margination*. They are then able to quickly flatten themselves and squeeze through the spaces between cells to reach the injury area – a process called *diapedesis*. Now at the injury site they attempt to destroy the invading microbes by phagocytosis. Macrophages arrive on the scene hours later and as the 'big eaters' engulf damaged tissue. Within a few days, a pocket of dead phagocytes and damaged tissue forms. This collection of dead cells and fluid is called *pus*. Pus formation usually continues until the infection has subsided.

Antimicrobial proteins enhance the innate defence mechanism by attacking micro-organisms directly or by hindering their ability to reproduce (Marieb & Hoehn, 2019). The most important antimicrobial proteins are *interferons* and *complement* proteins. Interferons are small proteins produced by some infected cells to protect cells that have not yet been infected. They stimulate nearby cells to synthesize protein that 'interferes' with viral replication. Complement or the complement system, refers to a group of 20 normally inactive proteins in blood plasma. They become activated in an orderly sequence by enzymes when an immune response is initiated and are a key weapon in the fight against infection. When activated, they enhance (complement) the immune, allergic and inflammatory reactions. Complement lyse micro-organisms enhance phagocytosis and intensify inflammatory and other immune responses (Marieb & Hoehn, 2019).

The adaptive defence mechanism is the body's built-in 'specific' defence mechanism. Unlike the innate system, which is always ready to spring into action, the adaptive system is triggered by an initial exposure to a foreign substance – an *antigen*, and this takes time. However, the adaptive mechanism is *specific*, it recognises and targets particular pathogens, it is *systemic*, immunity is not restricted to the infection site and it has *memory* – it recognises and mounts even stronger attacks on previously encountered pathogens. Your body is truly amazing!

An antigen is any chemical substance that when introduced into the body is recognised as foreign (Tortora & Derrickson, 2017). Antigens are also called *immunoglobulin*.

The specific immune system involves two types of lymphocytes developed in the bone marrow:

- *B lymphocytes (B cells)*
- *T lymphocytes (T cells)*

B lymphocytes work by a humoral type of immune response; this means that immunity is provided by antibodies present in the body's 'humors' (fluid) (Marieb & Hoehn, 2019). When lymphocytes themselves rather than the antibodies defend the body, this type of immune response is called *cellular* because the living cells provide the protection. T lymphocytes are an example of cellular immunity.

When an antigen invades the body it activates B lymphocyte cells. B lymphocytes have the ability to 'remember' antigens and make antibodies against them. Each B lymphocyte cell has proteins on their surface that are different membrane-bound antibodies. These antibodies bind specifically to an antigen, mounting a chemical attack on them, which marks the antigens for destruction by phagocytes or complement.

T lymphocytes can be broken down into two different types: helper T cells and cytotoxic T cells. B lymphocytes present the antigen to helper T cells. Helper T cells secrete cytokines (chemical messengers within the immune system) and these increase the production of the B lymphocytes antibody-mediated reaction by making them divide more quickly. Cytokines also activate destructive cytotoxic T cells. Cytotoxic T cells are the only T cells that can directly attack and kill other cells. Cytotoxic T cells are activated by antigens on the infected cell and secrete perforins that cause pores (holes) in the cell wall, resulting in the cell bursting.

PATHOPHYSIOLOGY: ACS AND SHOCK

ACS

Acute Coronary Syndrome (ACS) describes a spectrum of clinical conditions, including ST-segment myocardial infarction (*STEMI*), non ST-segment myocardial infarction (*NSTEMI*) and unstable angina (NICE, 2020). ACS is as an umbrella term for a group of conditions, which excludes stable angina. It can be viewed as a continuum with some patients' disease progression worsening from unstable angina to STEMI. ACS however is not a diagnosis in itself and can be divided into two main groups:

1. ST elevation myocardial infarction
2. Unstable angina and non ST elevation myocardial infarction

In order to understand pathophysiology of ACS it is necessary to be reminded of the blood supply to the heart, remembering that despite the many litres of blood that are pumped through the heart every minute, this is not where the heart draws its own blood supply from. The coronary arteries form a crown around the myocardium, the Latin term *corona* meaning crown. As the heart is an aerobic, constantly active organ, an efficient coronary circulation must provide a rich blood supply to the myocardium. A complex network of capillaries passes through the myocardium to the myocytes (Figure 6.6).

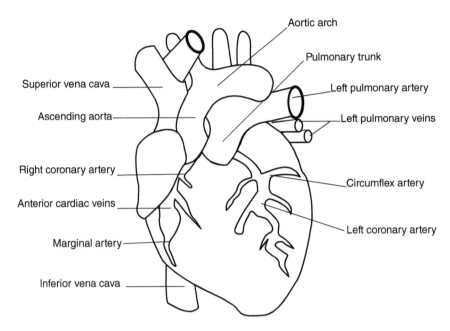

Figure 6.6   Coronary arteries

Blood supply to the heart is broadly divided into two coronary arteries: the right coronary artery (RCA) with the posterior descending artery branching from it; and the left coronary artery (LCA) with the circumflex artery wrapping itself around the base of the heart. In 85–90% of people the RCA is the dominant larger vessel because it supplies circulation to the inferior portion of the interventricular septum. Junctions between arteries, anastomoses, are key areas for potential artery disease in the mature heart as atheroma developing there renders a larger area of myocardium at risk.

Coronary heart disease and ACS occur due to the *atherosclerotic* process developing in the coronary arteries. Atherosclerotic plaque is a fat-laden inflammatory lesion caused by injury to the lining of the artery. It is more complex than the colloquial term of 'furring up of the arteries' often compared to the limescale deposition occurring in areas of hard water in the home. Atheroma formation is understood to develop in stages over decades (Figure 6.7).

Endothelial injury is thought to be the primary event in developing atherosclerosis and occurs due to physical or chemical forces within the artery damaging the intimal lining, which is a key protective mechanism within the artery. Over time, key risk factors such as hypertension with its rapid, turbulent blood flow and the resulting sheer forces damage the intimal layer. Smoking sees oxygen radicals damage the lining alongside potential high concentration of lipids such as cholesterol in the bloodstream contributed to by diet and obesity, causing injury and activating the immune system. All forms of injury reduce the effectiveness of the endothelium as a barrier.

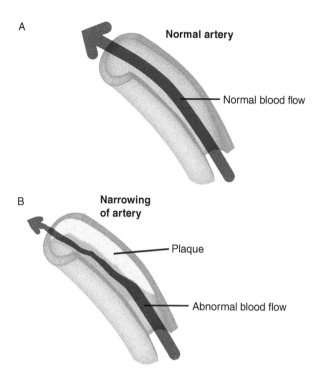

Figure 6.7 Stages of narrowing coronary artery and stages of atheroma formation

Fatty streaks are formed by infiltration of lipids, particularly low density lipoproteins (LDL) and white blood cells, into the lining of the coronary arteries, thought to be present in most people by the age of 20 but causing no symptoms. LDLs transform into foam cells, which form the fatty streaks; they result in yellow discolouration on the inner surface but do not protrude or impede blood flow and may regress over time. Over time a fibrous plaque develops consisting of collagen-rich sclerotic tissue with a thick fibrous cap over the thrombogenic lipid core. The plaque gradually increases in size and the vessel walls remodel to accommodate the deposition and preserve the diameter of the lumen. Collateral arteries are now known to develop to continue to supply the tissue with blood and oxygen. Even at this stage a patient can be free of symptoms as the heart adapts to the changing blood supply. Vulnerable plaques however are soft, have a larger fatty core and have a thin cap of fibrous tissue, which is prone to rupture if dislodged by turbulent rapid blood flow. If plaque rupture occurs, the highly thrombogenic contents will be exposed to the flowing blood activating platelet adhesion and aggregation, causing coagulation and thrombus development. Sometimes these thrombi can be small and are reabsorbed into the blood stream without causing damage; however if total occlusion occurs, oxygenated blood supply to the affected area of myocardium will cease and myocyte death will occur.

Shock

The term *shock* refers to a generalised severe reduction in blood supply to the body tissues. This inadequate tissue perfusion leads to cellular hypoxia and tissue damage. A good analogy for understanding the consequences of shock is to compare it to the functions of the domestic heating system. Shock results from the *pump* being unable to maintain adequate perfusion despite the constriction of the *pipes,* or if the *volume* is insufficient despite the attempt to increase the work of the pump and constrict the vessels, or if the pipes are too dilated for the volume available to fill an adequate pressure and for the pump to work effectively.

Shock can be classified into four categories according to the underlying cause:

- Hypovolaemic shock – reduction of circulating blood volume
- Cardiogenic shock – cardiac pump failure
- Obstructive shock – obstruction to blood flow
- Distributive shock – altered vascular resistance, which includes:
  - Anaphylactic
  - Septic
  - Neurogenic

Although the causes are varied the end results are the same at cellular level – cellular hypoxia and potential damage.

All body organs and tissues need a regular and consistent supply of oxygen for the metabolic waste products to be removed. This homeostatic regulation is maintained primarily by the cardiovascular system, which we considered earlier in the chapter. During shock, one or more of these components of cellular haemodynamics is disrupted:

- Cardiac Output (CO) – volume of blood pumped out per contraction (CO = SV x HR)
- Stroke Volume (SV) – amount of blood pumped into the aorta with each contraction
- Mean Arterial Pressure (MAP) = CO x SVR
- Systemic Vascular Resistance (SVR) – smooth muscle tone of arteries and arterioles (sympathetic tone)

Before considering the types of shock in more detail, the body's response to this insult on oxygen and nutrient delivery can be further classified into stages:

- Initial
- Compensatory/reversible
- Progressive/uncompensated
- Refractory/irreversible

Stages of shock comprise continuous and complex processes; there is usually no sudden transition from one stage to another. The process may take place over several hours or several days. The *initial response* to decreased tissue perfusion will vary and be dependent on the general state of health and presenting comorbidities as well as age. In the initial stages of shock, cellular changes are taking place in response to the disturbance in cellular perfusion and oxygenation. As the decreased tissue perfusion takes hold and the oxygen supply to the cells is depleted, cells switch to metabolising anaerobically (without oxygen). The by-product of this anaerobic metabolism is the production of lactic and pyruvic acid, which is damaging to the cells, damaging the cell membrane and the regulation of homeostatic mechanisms within the cell. This change in cellular metabolism and the development of metabolic acidosis emphasises the importance of measuring respiratory rate clinically as this may be the first and key indicator of deterioration in your patient. An increase in respiratory rate reflects this increased effort for oxygenation of the cells.

As the tissue perfusion continues to deteriorate and blood pressure is no longer able to adequately perfuse cells with oxygen and nutrients, a series of *compensatory* mechanisms are initiated. These compensatory mechanisms are referred to as the *compensatory stage of shock* or the *reversible stage*. This is a helpful reminder that if signs and symptoms are detected early and intervention is timely and appropriate, shock can be reversible. Neural compensatory measures are triggered due to hypotension. Baroreceptor reflexes are inhibited and cardioacceleratory functions are stimulated, causing an increase in myocardial contractility, tachycardia and vaso-constriction. This neural compensation also activates hormonal compensation. A fall in cardiac output will also impact on the renal system, which detects a decrease in blood flow and pressure to the kidneys. This initiates the renin-angiotensin-aldosterone mechanism considered earlier in the chapter and stimulates the adrenal cortex. The adrenal medulla secretes adrenaline and noradrenaline, which increases blood flow to the heart, meeting the oxygen demand. This stimulation of the fight or flight syndrome also contributes to improved cerebral perfusion and is responsible for the tachycardia. Aldosterone and anti-diuretic hormone release further contribute to the preservation of blood pressure by retention of fluid. A reduction in cardiac output also leads to a decrease in blood flow to the lungs detected by chemoreceptors in the aorta and carotid arteries. Chemoreceptors detect chemical change peripherally and centrally, responding to alteration in pH, oxygen, carbon dioxide and hydrogen levels. A reduction in carbon dioxide being 'blown off' impacts on blood flow and oxygen levels to the brain, which can lead to confusion and restlessness. This restlessness and agitation may be an early warning sign of decreased tissue perfusion and shock. This can lead to respiratory alkalosis. Detection by chemoreceptors leads to stimulation of the brain respiratory centre, increasing the rate and depth of ventilation, increasing expired carbon dioxide and raising blood pH.

The *progressive stage* of shock follows the compensatory stage. Compensatory mechanisms have failed to restore blood pressure and tissue perfusion. Impaired cellular metabolism occurs due to an inadequate blood supply of oxygen and nutrients, and decreased levels of oxygen. The cells now fully switch to functioning anaerobically. If the original problem is not corrected (e.g. haemorrhage), failure of the microcirculation will occur, increased capillary permeability and a movement of fluid from the interstitial space to the blood causing tissue dehydration will continue, thrombosis may develop as coagulation occurs, cellular dysfunction is pervasive and lactic acidosis destroys the cells.

The *refractory stage* of shock is irreversible. The continued decrease in blood pressure and heart rate means that the inadequate tissue perfusion leads to the subsequent failure of the body to respond to any form of therapy, which results in multi-system organ failure and death within a matter of hours.

Hypovolaemic shock

Hypovolaemic shock (*hypo* = below or deficient, *volaemia* = blood volume) is the most common type of shock. Hypovolaemic shock may be due to either an overt or occult haemorrhagic cause and leads to a reduction in circulating volume. A person who has experienced blood loss due to a puncture to the skin will have an overt loss of blood whereas a person experiencing bleeding internally will have an occult cause. Non-haemorrhagic causes of hypovolaemic shock include a person experiencing sepsis will have a hidden (occult) fluid loss as fluid shifts from the intra-cellular to the extracellular space, causing a relative hypovolaemia. Other non-haemorrhagic causes include severe burns, vomiting, diarrhoea and excessive diuresis. The reduction in circu-lating volume leads to a reduction in venous return and a resultant decrease in cardiac output. An imbalance develops between the body's demand for oxygen as fuel and the supply from decreasing amounts of oxygenated blood. This results in a switch from cells functioning aerobi-cally to *anaerobically* (without oxygen) with the by-product of lactic acid being produced.

Haemorrhage can be classified according to its origin as capillary, venous or arterial. The American College of Surgeons' classification of shock used as part of the Advanced Trauma Life support course (American College of Surgeons, 2018) provides some indication of the amount of blood loss and effect on corresponding vital signs observed with the four stages of shock numbered I, II, III and IV (see Table 6.1). There has been debate as to the usefulness of this tool in practice as presenting patient parameters may not fit into the categories identified, particu-larly the correlation between heart rate and systolic blood pressure and the underestimation of the degree of cognitive impairment (Mutschler et al., 2015). However, it can be a useful starting point and the classes broadly correlate to the stages of shock. As can be seen in the table, blood pressure is stable at first but eventually drops if blood loss continues. Hypotension is a late indicator of hypovolaemic shock and carries a poor prognosis as compensatory mechanisms are failing.

Table 6.1 Classification of hypovolaemic shock based on an average blood volume of 5 litres

	Class I	Class II	Class III	Class IV
Blood loss ml	Up to 750	750–1500	1500–2000	>2000
Blood loss (% blood volume)	<15	15–30	31–40	>40
Pulse rate	<100	100–120	120–140	>140
Blood pressure	Normal	Normal	Decreased	Decreased
Pulse pressure (mmHg)	Normal or increased	Decreased	Decreased	Decreased
Respiratory rate (per minute)	14–20	20–30	30–40	>35
Urine output (ml/hour)	>30	20–30	5–15	Negligible
Central nervous system/mental status	Slightly anxious	Mildly anxious	Anxious, confused	Confused, lethargic

Blood loss can be difficult to estimate in the presenting patient and is particularly complex when the bleeding is internal. A patient with a fractured shaft of femur can have an estimated blood and fluid loss of 2000ml, while a patient with a traumatic fracture of the tibia can lose an estimated 800ml into the surrounding tissue (Tait, 2016). In acute blood loss, blood should be replaced with blood rather than large volumes of crystalloid as this has the ability to promote clotting and carry oxygen. Balancing the goal of organ perfusion and tissue oxygenation with the avoidance of rebleeding by accepting a lower-than-normal blood pressure referred to as *permissive hypotension* may be a bridge to the surgical control of bleeding (American College of Surgeons, 2018). Tying together the presenting symptoms with an underpinning understanding of the mechanism of injury will help to identify risk and potential for deterioration.

Activity 6.4

A Massive Transfusion Protocol (MTP) should be used in critically bleeding patients anticipated to require massive transfusion.
    Identify the MTP for your clinical area.

Cardiogenic shock

Cardiogenic shock occurs when the heart fails to act effectively as a pump to maintain effective circulation. In most cases (up to 85%) this is caused by primary myocardial failure due to a myocardial infarction, often affecting the anterior surface of the heart muscle largely responsible for the force of contraction and systemic outflow. This reduces contractility of heart muscle, reduces stroke volume, which in turn reduces cardiac output and reduces blood pressure. As shock progresses myocardial workload increases (in an already failing heart), venous congestion occurs, leading to pulmonary oedema, tissue hypoxia and acidosis. Cardiac arrhythmia could further contribute to a failing pumping mechanism due to decreasing preload and increased workload of the heart. Myocardial contusions (bruising) often caused by or in combination with pericarditis can reduce movement of the ventricles and contribute to worsening cardiac performance. Cardiac tamponade, cardiomyopathy, valve disease and drug toxicity causing heart failure are additional causes.

Obstructive shock

Obstructive shock is sometimes excluded from classification as its causes and effects overlap other categories of shock, particularly cardiogenic shock. Obstructive shock is due to an obstruction to the circulating blood flow causing cardiomegaly, pulmonary oedema and jugular venous distention. All of these interfere with the ability of the heart to be able to pump effectively and affect blood pressure, heart rate and tissue perfusion with oxygen. Obstruction can be due to cardiac tamponade (*heart plug*) where inflammatory fluid seeps into the myocardial and pericardial layers of the heart. Obstruction could also be caused by a tension pneumothorax where air leaks into the pleural and thoracic cavity and causes an increase in pressure. Both of these causes mean the heart can no longer expand, the ventricles are squashed and blood has difficulty returning to the right atria and ventricle. A pulmonary embolism occluding the pulmonary vessels and ability of the heart to push blood out to the lungs to be re-oxygenated and return oxygenated blood to the left side of the heart is another cause.

Distributive shock

In *distributive shock*, the blood volume is normal but circulation is poor due to altered distribution of blood flow. A common cause of distributive shock is loss of vasomotor tone due to *anaphylaxis*. Anaphylaxis is a severe, life-threatening, generalised or systemic hypersensitivity reaction to drugs, toxins, foods or plants characterised by a rapid onset. *Immunoglobulin E (IgE)* is a type of antibody that is present in minute amounts in the body but plays a major role in allergic diseases. IgE binds to allergens and triggers the release of substances from mast cells that can cause inflammation. When IgE binds to mast cells, a cascade of allergic reaction begins. Initially, they cause profound vasodilation through the release of histamine and other vasodilatory mediators from mast cells and basophils and produce a relative hypovolaemia. This is due to increased vascular permeability and resulting capillary leakage, thereby reducing circulatory volume, venous return, preload, stroke volume and cardiac output. The tissues are hypoperfused and an acidotic state occurs. The allergic reaction produces some key identifiable symptoms and also a real danger in terms of patient mortality hence NICE (2011, updated 2020) and the Resuscitation Council (UK) (2008) guidance to treat anaphylaxis as a medical emergency.

Anaphylaxis causes around 20 deaths each year in the UK, although this may be an underestimate. Approximately 50% of fatalities are due to circulatory collapse (shock) and the rest are due to respiratory failure (asphyxia) (Resuscitation Council (UK), 2008).

Angioedema of the airway caused by the mast cell mediated allergic response can develop quickly and is life threatening. Tachypnoea, bronchoconstriction, wheezing and stridor occur due to inflammation of the airway along with skin changes such as erythema and urticaria. Anaphylaxis is likely when all of the following three criteria are met:

- Sudden onset and rapid progression of symptoms
- Life-threatening Airway and/or Breathing and/or Circulation problems
- Skin and/or mucosal changes (flushing, urticaria, angioedema) (Resuscitation Council (UK), 2008)

Sepsis is defined as a life-threatening organ dysfunction caused by a dysregulated host response to infection (Singer et al., 2016). Dysregulated means there is an impairment in the body's usual response to infection and the body's response to an infection injures its own tissues and organs. 'Septic shock should be defined as a subset of sepsis in which particularly profound circulatory, cellular, and metabolic abnormalities are associated with a greater risk of mortality than with sepsis alone' (Singer et al., 2016). NICE (2016, updated 2017) sepsis guidelines support this defining septic shock as persisting hypotension requiring vasopressors to maintain a mean arterial pressure (MAP) of 65 mmHg or more and having a serum lactate level of greater than 2 mmol/l despite adequate volume resuscitation. Singer et al. (2016) found that limitations of previous definitions included an excessive focus on inflammation, identified as a misleading model that sepsis follows a continuum through severe sepsis to shock, and inadequate specificity and sensitivity of the systemic inflammatory response syndrome (SIRS) criteria. The task force concluded that the term *severe sepsis* was redundant and new terminology suggests using the terms *sepsis* and *septic shock* only (NICE, 2016, updated 2017).

Infection occurs when normally sterile tissue, fluid or a body cavity is invaded by a pathogenic micro-organism. We have already considered the body's innate and adaptive immune response to infection. For some patients this infection can progress to sepsis; in patients who have unexplained organ dysfunction this should also raise the possibility of underlying sepsis. In sepsis this response becomes *dysregulated* or 'maladaptive' and organ dysfunction is present. In sepsis a complex series of physiological events occur simultaneously. Massive *cytokine* release is the initiator of these events and causes:

- Vasodilation and hypotension causing a reduction in tissue perfusion.
- Increased capillary permeability causing a mal-distribution of blood volume between the three fluid compartments (intracellular, intravascular and the interstitial); this will cause swelling, relative hypovolaemia and further hypo-perfusion and pain due to pressure on nerve endings.
- Inflammatory response and fever – redness and heat of the affected area.
- Endothelium dysfunction – microvascular endothelial damage from the invading pathogen and maladaption of the diapedesis process affects the ability of this lining of the blood vessels to maintain homeostasis.
- Activation of the clotting cascade.
- Renal, hepatic, respiratory and cardiac dysfunction.

The quick Sequential Organ Failure Assessment (qSOFA) tool recommended for assessing the degree of organ dysfunction will be considered in the next chapter.

Neurogenic shock reflects failure of the autonomic nervous system, which causes vasodilation of blood vessels and can be due to cervical spinal cord injury, anaesthesia, brain injury or sedation. It is rare and beyond the focus of this text.

Pathophysiology: Renal focusing on Acute Kidney Injury

Every day the kidneys filter nearly 200 litres of fluid from our bloodstream and have a key role in maintaining homeostatic balance in the body. As with many other body systems we are unappreciative of their function until something goes wrong. The main functions of the kidney include:

- Excretion of nitrogenous wastes: urea and creatinine
- Homeostatic control of water
- Homeostatic control of electrolytes
- Control of blood pressure
- Acid-base balance
- Erythropoiesis
- Vitamin D conversion to its activated form
- Calcium and phosphate homeostasis
- Excretion of drugs and toxins (Donald, 2011)

The functional unit of the kidney is the nephron with its primary function of filtration (not the production of urine). Key to the roles of the kidney are the three processes involved in the formation of urine:

- Glomerular filtration
- Tubular reabsorption
- Tubular secretion

Activity 6.5

Review your understanding of these three processes.

These normal processes can be reviewed in an anatomy and physiology text in order to inform understanding of a syndrome now referred to as Acute Kidney Injury (AKI) (previously acute renal failure). Detection of Acute Kidney Injury is focused on changes in urine output and blood chemistry, particularly monitoring of serum creatinine levels (KDIGO, 2012; NICE, 2019b). The *glomerular filtration rate* (GFR) is widely accepted as the best overall index of kidney function in health and disease. However, GFR is difficult to measure and is commonly estimated from the serum level of filtration markers, such as creatinine (KDIGO, 2012). *Creatinine* is a waste product from metabolised protein ingested or from muscle injury. The normal creatinine range is 60–120 µmol/L. A raised serum creatinine level means kidney damage although it should be noted that creatinine levels tend to be higher in men and people with large muscles. *Blood Urea Nitrogen* (BUN) is another measure of wastes (urea) in the blood produced from the metabolism of protein. A high BUN level usually means that kidney function is less than normal, but other factors may affect the BUN level such as bleeding in the intestines or dehydration.

In adults, acute kidney injury can be detected by using any of the following criteria:

- A rise in serum creatinine of 26 µmol/L or greater within 48 hours.
- A 50% or greater rise in serum creatinine known or presumed to have occurred within the past seven days.
- A fall in urine output to less than 0.5ml/kg/hour for more than six hours (NICE, 2019b).

KDIGO (2012) recommend that early detection and treatment of AKI may improve outcomes. Two similar definitions based on serum creatinine and urine output (RIFLE and AKIN) have been proposed and validated. The severity of AKI was first classified by Bellomo, Kellum and Ronco (2012) and referred to as the RIFLE criteria (Risk, Injury, Failure, Loss and End Stage Kidney Disease). The criteria help to identify people who have renal impairment and are at risk, as well as those with injury. Later work by the Acute Kidney Injury Network (AKIN) modified these to increase sensitivity and specificity of diagnosis. KDIGO (2012) combined this classification, summarised in Table 6.2, which demonstrates the progression of deteriorating kidney function. The inclusion of urine output is useful when baseline creatinine is unknown.

Staging of AKI

Table 6.2   Stages of Acute Kidney Injury

Stage	Criteria
1 (Risk)	Serum creatinine 1.5–1.9 times baseline
	Urine output <0.5ml/kg/h for 6–12 hours
2 (Injury)	Serum creatinine 2.0–2.9 times baseline
	Urine output <0.5ml/kg/h for ≥ 12 hours
3 (Failure)	Serum creatinine 3.0 times baseline
	Urine output <0.3ml/kg/h for ≥ 24 hours or Anuria for ≥ 12 hours

Acute Kidney Injury occurs as a result of volume depletion and hypoperfusion to the kidneys, decreased renal blood flow and/or toxic inflammatory injury to the kidneys (Tait & Hanson, 2016). AKI may be:

- Pre-renal (volume responsive)
- Intra-renal (or intrinsic)
- Post-renal

Pre-renal AKI (occurring *before* the kidneys) is due to hypoperfusion of the kidneys resulting from reduced blood volume, for example as occurs in shock considered earlier. A decrease in blood volume and blood pressure will mean there is less fluid filtering through the glomerulus in the kidneys due to stimulation of the renin-angiotensin-aldosterone mechanism. Pre-renal AKI is also referred to as *volume responsive*, indicating that if the underlying cause of the reduced perfusion is identified and corrected then the risk of injury is reversible. For example, if fluid resuscitation is undertaken in a timely and appropriate manner, the risk of injury can be halted and reversed. *Intra-renal AKI* (occurring within the kidney) occurs due to the interruption in blood supply, damaging the tissues leading to ischaemia and *acute tubular necrosis* (ATN). The longer the interruption in blood supply, the greater the potential for injury. As well as the reduction in blood supply, ATN can also be caused by nephrotoxic damage to the kidney from inhaling or ingesting toxic chemicals or from a hypersensitivity reaction, for example to antibiotics or radiographic contrast.

Common ATN causing antibiotics are:

- Gentamicin
- Vancomycin
- Rifampicin
- Ciprofloxacin

In addition, non-steroidal anti-inflammatory drugs (NSAIDS) such as Diclofenac and Angiotensin Converting Enzyme (ACE) Inhibitors, such as Ramipril, are also nephrotoxic.

In ATN, damaged epithelium allows filtrate to leak through the membranes and be reabsorbed into the circulation. Debris from red blood cells, damaged cells and cellular debris will build up in the tissue and prevent the flow of filtrate. Ischaemic damage to the epithelial cells reduces their permeability and damages the capillary endothelium. Fluid seeps from the capillaries into the tissues and causes cellular swelling and tubular obstruction. Ischaemic damage results in deep lesions to the tubular epithelium and basement membrane – this damage is permanent. Nephrotoxic injury causes damage to the epithelium; however the basement membrane remains intact – this is reversible.

Post renal AKI (occurring *after* the kidney) results from bilateral obstruction of urine output. This may be due to:

- Enlarged prostate
- Tumour
- Stones in urinary tract
- Urethral strictures

These require urological intervention and will not be a focus in discussion within this text.

SUMMARY

This chapter has presented the anatomy and physiology of the cardiovascular system. The workings of the systemic and pulmonary circuit have been explored along with understanding of how the mechanical events of contraction link with electrical activity. Physiological regulation of fluid balance, the immune response and thermoregulation have been considered. These normal processes have been applied to development of acute coronary syndrome, shock, acute kidney injury, sepsis and anaphylaxis. The following chapter will apply this understanding by considering the assessment and management of the patient with these conditions.

REFERENCES

American College of Surgeons (2018) *Advanced Trauma Life Support (ATLS)* (10th ed.), Student Course Manual. Chicago: American College of Surgeons. Available at: https://viaaerearcp. files.wordpress.com/2018/02/atls-2018.pdf (accessed 3 January 2020).

Arrich, J., Holzer, M., Havel, C., Müllner, M. & Herkner, H. (2016) *Hypothermia for neuroprotection in adults after cardiopulmonary resuscitation.* Cochrane Database of Systematic Reviews [online], 2 (CD004128). Available at: http://cochranelibrary-wiley.com/doi/10.1002/14651858.CD004128. pub4/full (accessed 12 June 2018).

Bellomo, R., Kellum, J. & Ronco, C. (2012) Acute kidney injury. *Lancet*, 380, 756–766.

Donald, R. (2011) Caring for the renal system. In M. Macintosh & T. Moore (Eds.), *Caring for the Seriously Ill Patient* (2nd ed.) (pp. 73–97). London: Hodder Arnold.

Kidney Disease: Improving Global Outcomes (KDIGO) Acute Kidney Injury Work Group (2012) KDIGO clinical practice guideline for Acute Kidney Injury. *Kidney International Supplements*, 2, 1–138.

Marieb, E. & Hoehn, K. (2019) *Human Anatomy and Physiology* (11th ed.). London: Pearson.

Mutschler, M., Hoffman, M., Wolfl, C., Münzberg, M., Schipper, I., Paffrath, T., Bouillon, B. & Maegele, M. (2015) Is the ATLS classification of hypovolaemic shock appreciated in daily trauma care? An online-survey among 383 ATLS course directors and instructors. *Emergency Medicine Journal*, 32, 134–137.

Nolan, J., Deakin, C., Lockey, A., Perkins, G. & Soar, J. (2015) *Post-resuscitation care.* Available at: www.resus.org.uk/resuscitation-guidelines/post-resuscitation-care/ (accessed 12 June 2018).

NICE (2011, updated 2020) *Anaphylaxis: Assessment and referral after emergency treatment.* Cg134. Available at: https://test.nice.org.uk/guidance/cg134/resources/anaphylaxis-assessment-and-referral-after-emergency-treatment-pdf-35109510368965 (accessed 25 January 2022).

NICE (2016, updated 2017) *Sepsis: Recognition, diagnosis and early management.* Ng51. Available at: www.nice.org.uk/guidance/NG51 (accessed 25 January 2022).

NICE (2019a) *Hypertension in adults: Diagnosis and management.* Ng136. Available at: www. nice.org.uk/guidance/ng136/resources/hypertension-in-adults-diagnosis-and-management-pdf-66141722710213 (accessed 25 January 2022).

NICE (2019b) *Acute kidney injury: Prevention, detection and management.* Ng 148. Available at: www.nice.org.uk/guidance/ng148/resources/acute-kidney-injury-prevention-detection-and-management-pdf-66141786535621 (accessed 25 January 2022).

NICE (2020) *Acute coronary syndromes.* Ng185. Available at: www.nice.org.uk/guidance/NG185 (accessed 25 January 2022).

Resuscitation Council (UK) (2008) *Emergency Treatment of Anaphylactic Reactions: Guidelines for Healthcare Providers.* Working Group of the Resuscitation Council (UK).

Singer, M., Deutschman, C., Seymour, C., Shankar-Hari, M., Annane, D., Bauer, M,, Bellomo, R., Bernard, G., Chiche, J., Coopersmith, C., Hotchkiss, R., Levy, M., Marshall, J., Martin, G., Opal, S., Rubenfeld, G., van der Poll, T., Vincent, J. & Angus, D. (2016) The third international consensus definitions for sepsis and septic shock (sepsis-3). *JAMA*, 3415 (8), 801–810.

Tait, D. (2016) The patient in shock. In D. Tait, J. James, C. Williams & D. Barton (Eds.), *Acute and Critical Care in Adult Nursing* (2nd ed.) (pp. 122–146). London: Sage.

Tait, D. & Hanson, S. (2016) The patient with acute kidney injury. In D. Tait, J. James, C. Williams & D. Barton (Eds.), *Acute and Critical Care in Adult Nursing* (2nd ed.). London: Sage.

Tortora, G. & Derrickson, B. (2017) *Principles of Anatomy and Physiology*. New York: Wiley.

World Health Organisation (WHO) (2018) The top 10 causes of death. Available at: www.who.int/news-room/fact-sheets/detail/the-top-10-causes-of-death (accessed 3 January 2020).

7
PATIENT-CENTRED APPROACHES TO CIRCULATION: APPLICATION TO PRACTICE

ALICE SKULL

Chapter learning outcomes

By the end of this chapter you will be able to:

1. Understand how to systematically assess a patient experiencing difficulties with their circulatory system.
2. Describe the signs and symptoms of acute coronary syndrome and cardiogenic shock, sepsis, hypovolaemia, Acute Kidney Injury (AKI) and anaphylaxis.
3. Understand the management of the patient experiencing difficulties with their circulatory system, identifying key national drivers.
4. Explain the impact on the patient and family, and strategies to support them.

Key words

- Acute coronary syndrome
- Cardiogenic shock
- Sepsis
- Hypovolaemia
- Acute Kidney Injury
- Anaphylaxis

INTRODUCTION

This chapter will present five case studies of patients who are experiencing difficulties with their circulatory system. For each case study, an initial assessment will take place to identify and prioritise the patients' key problems. Application of previously discussed pathophysiology will then be explored followed by evidence-based interventions and management strategies for each of the five case studies. The case studies will focus on: acute coronary syndrome and cardiogenic shock, sepsis, hypovolaemia, AKI and anaphylaxis.

CASE STUDY 7.1: ACUTE CORONARY SYNDROME AND CARDIOGENIC SHOCK – ANDY WEBB

Case study 7.1 takes a look at a patient with an acute coronary syndrome (ACS). According to the British Heart Foundation (2018) coronary heart disease (CHD) remains the single biggest cause of death in the UK, making it a key area for healthcare professionals to understand, assess and manage in a timely and appropriate manner. CHD is responsible for over 66,000 deaths each year in the UK, although mortality rates have fallen by 73% between 1974 and 2013, largely due to advancements in disease management both interventional and pharmacological. Over 97,000 percutaneous coronary interventions (PCIs) were carried out in 2015, more than two times higher than a decade ago. Together with increased numbers of patients surviving out of hospital cardiac arrest (OHCA), the morbidity statistics reveal increasing numbers of patients with coronary heart disease and an increased burden on hospital and community services to manage these patients.

It is not possible to differentiate the type of ACS purely by symptom presentation; indeed patients may present with the same symptoms but have different diagnoses. Key to identification of ACS is assessment of chest pain (NICE, 2010, updated 2016).

A summary of Andy's observations on reporting chest pain during the night are presented in Box 7.1.

Box 7.1 Andy's initial assessment

Mr Andy Webb is 57 years old and works in the City of London in finance. He was admitted with unstable angina. At 2am he calls you over, complaining of severe pressure in his chest and pain radiating to his lower jaw. He tells you that the pain is excruciating. He feels cold to the touch, dizzy and his bed is saturated with sweat. The pain has been increasing over the last 25 minutes.

Andy is married with two adult daughters. He weighs 83 kg.

(Continued)

Airway

- Andy is able to speak in full sentences; he says that his chest hurts

Breathing

- Respiratory rate: 21 breaths per minute (bpm)
- Oxygen saturation levels: 92% on air
- Chest clear on examination

Circulation

- Blood pressure: 100/50 mmHg
- Heart rate: 110 beats per minute, Sinus Tachycardia
- Temperature: 37°C
- Urine output: 65, 50 and 42 mls/hour over the past three hours
- Capillary refill time (CRT): 2 seconds
- ECG shows ST elevation leads V2–V6

Disability

- Alert on ACVPU
- Pain score 3/3, complaining of central chest pain radiating to lower jaw
- Blood glucose: 7.0 mmol/l

Acute Coronary Syndrome

Andy's presentation of chest pain radiating to his jaw and an electrocardiograph (ECG) indicating ST segment elevation indicate a diagnosis of ACS, specifically myocardial infarction. Determining whether the chest pain is cardiac in origin will involve considering the history of the chest pain, the presence of cardiovascular risk factors, history of heart disease and any previous investigations for chest pain. Patients experiencing chest pain indicative of ACS can describe it as occurring centrally in the chest, to be crushing or 'band-like' in nature or similar to severe indigestion. ACS should be suspected where chest pain lasts longer than 15 minutes (NICE, 2010, updated 2016). Comprehensive assessment should note the location, character, any radiation, exacerbating or relieving factors, duration, frequency and associated symptoms. Radiation of pain to the arms, jaw, back and shoulders can occur because of the shared neural pathway experiencing pressure from the damaged myocardium.

Other symptoms associated with chest pain and ACS are:

- Nausea and vomiting ⎤
- Sweating   ⎬ particularly in combination
- Breathlessness   ⎦
- Haemodynamic instability – hypotension, tachycardia, oliguria

The psychological impact of chest pain and the fear and anxiety that a patient can experience should not be underestimated, and can contribute to the clinical assessment and professional judgement in assessment and diagnosis.

Healthcare professionals should always be alert to atypical presentation of ACS particularly what is referred to as a 'silent MI' in patients who have diabetes or are older and have multiple comorbidities, making assessment and diagnosis more challenging. These groups of patients may present with epigastric pain, cardiac arrhythmias or vaguer symptoms of fatigue. NICE (2010, updated 2016) guidelines note that ACS symptoms should not be assessed differently in men and women, or amongst different ethnic groups and that response to Glyceryl Trinitrate (GTN) should not be used to make a diagnosis.

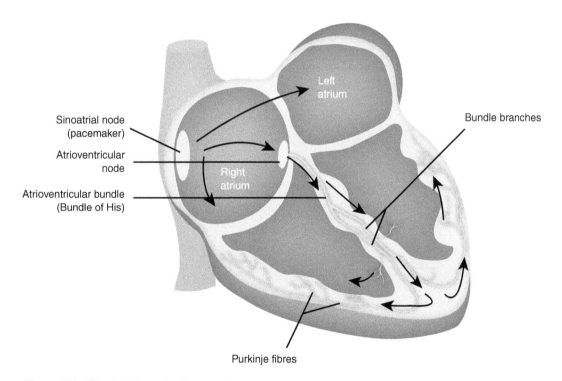

Figure 7.1 Electrical conduction system

NICE (2010, updated 2016) guidelines make it clear that management of ACS should start as soon as it is suspected, but should not delay transfer to hospital. Assessment and intervention is often initiated by the ambulance service. Development of ACS is a medical emergency and requires intervention in a timely and appropriate manner.

Andy's 12-lead ECG was taken as soon as possible and interpreted appropriately. This required some understanding of the electrical conduction system of the heart (Figure 7.1).

The heart works under electrical innervation with the Sino Atrial (SA) node setting the pace. The SA node is a bundle of specialised conducting fibres that have the intrinsic ability to depolarise and maintain a regular heart beat. It is located in the right atrium and normally fires between 60–100bpm. It sends its electrical impulse across the right and left atria via the Bachmann's bundle to the atrioventricular (AV) node. The activity of the SA node is represented by the 'p' wave on the ECG, a small, rounded, upright waveform (see Figure 7.2). The AV node holds that impulse for a short while before it travels down the Bundle of His to the right and left bundle branches, depolarising the ventricles with the electrical wave moving across the septum from the left to the right. The left bundle branch has two fascicles due to the increased muscle bulk on the left side and the need for the heart to contract as one functional unit – a syncytium. The Purkinje fibres ensure that the electrical wave reaches the outermost aspects of the myocardium. Depolarisation of the ventricles is represented on the ECG by the QRS complex with the T wave representing repolarisation of the ventricles (see Figure 7.2). Atrial repolarisation is masked by the QRS waveform.

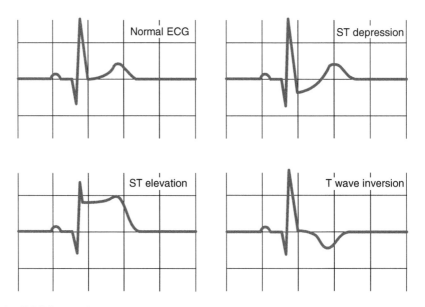

Figure 7.2   PQRS waveform

Pathophysiology

Diagnosis of ACS focuses on the ST segment and identification of ischaemic changes. Elevation of the ST segment from the isoelectric line occurs in full thickness myocardial infarction (STEMI) due to the necrosed area of myocardium creating an 'electrical window'. The recording electrode cannot record electrical activity travelling towards it. A diagnosis of STEMI is made where there is >1 mm ST elevation in two adjacent limb leads (I, II, III, aVR, aVL, aVF) or >2 mm in two adjacent chest leads (V1–V6).

The differing measurements required are due to the difference in amplitude of leads. Location of infarct can be labelled by description of the surface of the myocardium affected and some inference made as to which coronary artery is occluded. For example, an inferior STEMI is likely to be due to occlusion of the right coronary artery. New occurrence of a left bundle branch block should also be presumed to be indicative of myocardial infarction.

The unstable angina and NSTEMI ECG is usually abnormal. It can manifest itself as T wave and ST segment changes. The most common indications of myocardial ischaemia are ST depression and T wave inversion (see Figure 7.2).

A diagnosis of NSTEMI indicates a partial thickness of the myocardial wall is necrosed. A diagnosis of unstable angina indicates narrowing of the coronary arteries but without significant necrosis of the myocardium having occurred. Both diagnoses place the patient at risk of progressing onto a full thickness STEMI and at risk of deterioration.

Troponin is a cardiac biochemical marker used in diagnosis of ACS. Troponin is a protein attached to actin, the thin filament of the myofibril, which together with the thick filament myosin shortens and is responsible for muscle contraction. The Troponin complex is made up of three sub units, Troponin T, C and I. Troponin is not normally present in the blood stream but can be released as a result of damage to the myocytes' cell membrane caused by ischaemia. Troponin levels peak 6–12 hours after onset of acute MI and can be detected in the bloodstream for up to 14 hours post event. NICE (2010) recommends measuring a baseline Troponin on admission and a second 10–12 hours after symptom onset. Troponin is cardiac specific but not selective to MI. Other cardiac causes can elevate Troponin, for example heart failure, myocarditis and renal failure.

Management of Acute Coronary Syndrome

Management of ACS in the UK is driven by two clinical drivers: NICE NG 185 (NICE, 2020) and NICE CG 95 (NICE, 2010, updated 2016).

Assessment

Following on from the initial set of observations that were carried out, a National Early Warning Score (2) (Royal College of Physicians [RCP], 2017) was calculated for Andy. This found Andy had a high NEWS2 score of 7, which necessitated immediate referral to a specialist registrar and emergency response team such as the critical care outreach team (RCP, 2017). This was because Andy was at risk of rapid deterioration.

Whilst the nurse caring for Andy was contacting the critical care outreach team and cardiology registrar using an SBAR approach, she asked another nurse to implement continuous monitoring of vital signs including repeating an ECG every 15 minutes (RCP, 2017; NICE, 2020). This was done concurrently with no delay as the nurse had a high suspicion that Andy was having a myocardial infarction.

Box 7.2 SBAR handover to cardiology registrar and critical care outreach team

Situation, Background, Assessment, Recommendation (SBAR) (NHS Improvement, 2018)

S: I am Alice, a registered nurse on Ward A. I am calling about Andy Webb. I am calling because I am concerned that Andy has severe chest pain (3/3), he has a sinus tachycardia and his ECG shows ST elevation in leads V2–V6, his respiratory rate is 21bpm, oxygen saturation 92% on air and his blood pressure is 100/50 mmHg. His NEWS2 is 7.

B: Andy was admitted yesterday with unstable angina and reported chest pain at 2am. His previous observations at 22.00 were within normal parameters.

A: I think Andy is having a myocardial infarction and I have administered emergency oxygen and glyceryl trinitrate spray 2 puffs with no effect on the chest pain.

R: I need you to come and see the patient immediately. Would you like me to administer an antiplatelet and opioid analgesic in the meantime?

Ongoing management

Treatment for ACS needs to be started quickly with specific tasks to restore blood flow, reduce cardiac oxygen demands, reduce or treat complications and to ensure rapid access to resuscitation facilities. Within 15 minutes of vessel occlusion, myocytes death begins; 50% of myocardium at risk has died within 3 hours and 80% of myocardium at risk is permanently damaged by 12 hours (Zeitz & Quinn, 2010). Immediate assessment of eligibility for coronary reperfusion therapy should be made (NICE, 2020).

Coronary angiography with follow-on primary percutaneous coronary intervention (PPCI) should be offered for people with acute STEMI if presentation is within 12 hours of onset of symptoms and primary PCI can be delivered within 120 minutes of the time when fibrinolysis could have been given. Coronary angiography involves taking X-rays of the heart's arteries. Percutaneous coronary intervention, also referred to as *angioplasty*, is a procedure used to treat narrowed or occluded coronary arteries. A catheter with a small balloon at the end is inserted through an artery and the balloon is directed to the blockage using X-ray guidance. The balloon is then inflated so that it pushes the fatty tissue in the narrow artery out of the way in order to improve the blood supply in the heart. A metal stent inside the catheter expands as the balloon is inflated and allows the narrowed blood vessel to be enlarged and held in place. The balloon is then deflated and removed, leaving the stent in place; a process often called 'coronary stenting'.

Antiplatelet agents should be administered to prevent platelet aggregation and activation. The ISIS 2 (Baigent et al., 1998) trial demonstrated significant reduction in mortality for patients receiving a loading dose of Aspirin 300 mg and therefore this has become a mainstay of the ACS pathway along with further antiplatelet loading of Clopidogrel or alternative.

Chest pain should be assessed and managed with opioid analgesia such as IV Diamorphine being recommended. The BNF (2022) indicate a slow intravenous dose of 5 mg, followed by 2.5–5 mg if required, dose to be administered at a rate of 1–2 mg/minute. (For frail patients experiencing myocardial infarction the dose should be reduced.) Diamorphine does reduce blood pressure, slows heart rate, and relieves anxiety, which makes the patient feel better and may decrease myocardial oxygen demand. However, it also depresses respiration, which may decrease oxygenation and therefore needs to be carefully observed for its effects. Treatment of actual or potential nausea as a side effect of opioid analgesia should also be addressed. The vaso-dilator Glyceryl Trinitrate (GTN) may be a first choice. Due to its extensive first pass metabolism, it is unsuitable for oral use and administered sublingually as a spray in the acute phase. GTN releases nitric oxide in vascular smooth muscle target tissues and causes vasodilation, reduces preload and oxygen demand of the myocardium. This dilation of the coronary arteries may pro-vide some pain relief but commonly causes headaches due to cerebral vasodilation.

Andy was in a hospital facility that provides primary percutaneous coronary intervention (PPCI). On review by the cardiology team, he was immediately prepared for transfer to the PPCI unit having received a loading dose of 300mg Aspirin and Clopidogrel. The nurse administered the prescribed Diamorphine, titrating this to his pain accompanied by an anti-emetic, to enable him to be as pain-free as possible. Ongoing chest pain is an indication of the continuance of coronary artery occlusion. Oxygen was continued and titrated to achieve a target saturation of 94–98% in line with BTS (2017) guidance, via a venturi mask.

Debate around the use of oxygen in myocardial ischaemia was highlighted in the publica-tion of the *British Thoracic Guidelines for Emergency Oxygen Use* in 2008. Updated guidelines in 2017 highlighted that most patients with acute coronary artery syndromes are not hypoxaemic and the benefits/harms of oxygen therapy are unknown in such cases. Unnecessary use of high concentration oxygen may increase infarct size (BTS, 2017). Oxygen is a treatment for hypoxaemia and should be used to achieve target SpO_2 94–98% in adults not at risk of hypercapnic respiratory failure. In the case of non-hypoxaemic patients, it is not known if supplementary oxygen may be beneficial by increasing the amount of oxygen delivered to the hypoxaemic area of myocardium or whether it may actually cause vasoconstriction with increased systemic vascular resistance and reduced myocardial oxygen supply with worsened systolic myocardial performance. There is some evidence of potential harm due to reduced coronary blood flow and exacerbation of reperfusion injury to the heart, and a significantly greater rise in myocardial enzyme suggesting a greater infarct size has been linked to routine use of supplementary oxygen in myocardial infarction (O'Driscoll et al., 2008).

Andy's nurse carefully explained the plan of care and treatment to him and his family, taking care not to overload them with information. Development of this therapeutic relationship is key in reducing and managing anxiety for the patient and family. Completion of a pre-PPCI checklist aided this process.

Watch the video of the cardiology team at the Essex Cardiothoracic Centre, part of the Basildon and Thurrock University Hospitals NHS Foundation Trust outlining the techniques employed in the successful diagnosis and treatment of a myocardial infarction.

Activity 7.1

Watch this video from the Essex Cardiothoracic Centre designed to help healthcare professionals have confidence in referring a patient to a heart attack centre: www.youtube.com/watch?v=xIIMNry6SuO&t=338s

Andy underwent PPCI within 120 minutes of the onset of his symptoms and had coronary stenting to two of his coronary arteries. He was transferred to the cardiac ward to recover with the intention of discharging him after 48 hours. However, during the following evening, Andy's condition deteriorates – he struggles to maintain his blood pressure, reports feeling breathless with ongoing chest tightness.

Box 7.3 Andy's reassessment following PPCI

Airway

- Andy is able to speak in full sentences; he says he feels very unwell

(Continued)

Breathing

- Respiratory rate: 26 breaths per minute (bpm)
- Oxygen saturation levels: 91%
- Chest clear on examination

Circulation

- Blood pressure: 90/50 mmHg
- Heart rate: 125 beats per minute, Sinus Tachycardia
- Temperature: 37°C
- Urine output: 42, 25 and 7 mls/hour over the past three hours
- Capillary refill time (CRT): 4 seconds
- ECG shows resolving ST elevation leads V2–V6, Q waves developing

Disability

- Alert on ACVPU
- Pain score 2/3, complaining of chest tightness
- Blood glucose: 9.0 mmol/l

Exposure

- Pressure areas intact
- Skin cool and clammy to touch

Andy's NEWS2 (RCP, 2017) has increased to 13, indicating a deteriorating picture requiring an emergency response. The nurse initiated an SBAR call in light of the ABCDE assessment and because she had a high suspicion that Andy was developing signs of cardiogenic shock. Cardiogenic shock is the leading cause of death in acute myocardial infarction and develops in 7–10% of cases with mortality over 80% (Caceres et al., 2014).

Management

Airway and breathing

Indications are that Andy's airway remains patent as he is able to speak in full sentences. However, he reports difficulty in breathing and his respiratory rate has risen to 26 breaths per minute, the tachypnoea driven by chemoreceptor activity stimulating the sympathetic nervous system to compensate for the increase in metabolic demand. A falling oxygen saturation indicates compensation is failing and the body's demand is more than the supply – this is called 'cellular hypoxia'. High flow oxygen is recommended via a non-breathe mask at 15 litres/min (BTS, 2017). Andy is sat upright in bed to optimise his ventilation and reduce his oxygen demand. Blood was taken to measure the arterial blood gas. The high NEWS2 score initiated referral to the critical care outreach team and together with the cardiology team, consideration of the need for continuous positive airway pressure or endotracheal ventilation can be undertaken (see Chapter 3 for further detail on airway management).

Circulation

Another indication that compensation is failing is that Andy's blood pressure has fallen to 90/50 mmHg. Myocardial infarction causes significant reduction in the cardiac contractility, and a subsequent reduction in stroke volume, cardiac output and blood pressure. In this case Andy's cardiac output has deteriorated due to impaired myocardial performance and his myocardium cannot produce an adequate cardiac output. Andy's heart rate has increased in an attempt to improve performance and contractility, and compensatory mechanisms have led to a decreased capillary refill time of 4s (normal <2s) as blood is drawn away from the peripheries, vessels vasoconstrict and tissue perfusion decreases. Andy's hypotension has stimulated the renin-angiotensin-aldosterone system, leading to vasoconstriction, a decrease in urine output and electrolyte loss from the body. Andy's heart is developing pump failure as a result of the ischaemic and necrosed myocardium and is struggling to cope with the additional fluid volume being retained by the kidneys.

Andy needs continuous monitoring of his blood pressure, cardiac rhythm, pulse, respiratory rate, oxygen saturation and skin. Strict fluid balance monitoring needs to be continued and care of his urinary catheter. As Andy has signs of pump failure (cardiogenic shock), any intravenous fluid to be administered needs to be carefully evaluated as to how his heart will cope with the added volume. Blood should be taken to monitor electrolyte levels particularly focusing on sodium, potassium, magnesium and calcium in respect of his heart contractility and urea and creatinine to monitor his kidney function as he is at risk of AKI. Troponin levels should also be repeated to rule out re-infarction.

An echocardiogram (ultrasound) will be helpful to review the structure and function of Andy's heart and this can be done at the bedside by skilled practitioners.

Tissue perfusion needs to be optimised and review from the cardiology team should be sought immediately in respect of further invasive or mechanical circulatory support such as a ventricular assist device (VAD) or extracorporeal membrane oxygenation (ECMO) (Caceres et al., 2014).

Although evidence from clinical trials is limited regarding the use of vasopressor agents and inotropic support they may be of value to Andy as a bridge to more definitive support. Indeed, a recent systematic review by Léopold et al. (2018) identified a threefold increase in the risk of mortality in cardiogenic shock with the use of epinephrine. Epinephrine increases oxygen consumption and alters calcium homeostasis, a key mineral influencing cardiac contractility. In Andy's already severely compromised heart function, use of epinephrine could markedly aggravate cardiac metabolism leading to death. An alternative to support Andy's blood pressure would be norepinephrine, which is considered safer than dopamine and vasopressin (Mebazaa et al., 2018). Dobutamine would be a first choice for a predominantly low cardiac output and preserved perfusion pressure (Mebazaa et al., 2018). This would necessitate Level 2 care (Intensive Care Society, 2021) and risk assessment of the skill mix required to look after Andy is required.

Disability

Andy has reported experiencing chest tightness (2/3); his hypotension makes GTN an unsuitable choice, therefore diamorphine and an anti-emetic should be administered and titrated to his pain until he is pain free. Regular reassessment of pain or chest tightness should occur, always accompanied by repeating a 12-lead ECG.

ACVPU needs to be undertaken with the NEWS2 scoring. This will demonstrate how effective Andy's cerebral perfusion is. Blood glucose levels need to be monitored to evaluate the sympathetic nervous system (SNS) response to this acute illness. In times of physiological stress, the SNS will mobilise glucose through glycogenolysis to ensure there is adequate glucose available for cellular respiration. Andy's blood glucose is slightly elevated at 9 mmol/l (normal value 4–7 mmol/l); however intervention with sliding scale insulin is unlikely to commence at this level.

Exposure

At all times, Andy's pressure areas should be assessed. With his reduced mobility, poor peripheral perfusion, cool and clammy skin, Andy is at high risk of developing pressure ulcers. Interventions such as a pressure relieving mattress should be immediately implemented and a regular change of position and skin inspection.

A compassionate and caring approach towards Andy and his family needs to be taken, offering clear and honest explanation about the care provided. Reassurance, emotional and psychological support are key facets of the nurse's role for Andy in order to provide dignified and respectful care, upholding nursing values (Cummings & Bennett, 2012). In light of the high mortality rate for cardiogenic shock, the nursing team caring for Andy and his family will require this compassionate approach to discuss resuscitation in the event of cardiac arrest. Advance care planning and end of life issues are considered further in Chapter 9.

Conclusion

A case study considering a patient, Andy Webb presenting with an ACS progressing to cardiogenic shock has been considered, outlining the relevant pathophysiology and incorporating evidence-based interventions and management strategies.

CASE STUDY 7.2: SEPSIS – MARY NORTON

The second case study in this chapter looks at a patient who has developed sepsis. Sepsis is a clinical syndrome caused by the body's immune and coagulation systems being switched on by an infection (NICE, 2016a, updated 2017). Sepsis with shock is a life-threatening condition that is characterised by low blood pressure despite adequate fluid replacement, and organ dysfunction or failure. Sepsis is an important cause of death in people of all ages. The WHO (2018) estimate that sepsis affects more than 30 million people worldwide every year, potentially leading to six million deaths. Both a UK Parliamentary and Health Service Ombudsman enquiry (2013) (*Time to Act: Severe sepsis rapid diagnosis and treatment saves lives*) and a UK National Confidential Enquiry into Patient Outcome and Death (NCEPOD, 2015) (*Just say sepsis!*) highlighted sepsis as being a leading cause of avoidable death that kills more people than breast, bowel and prostate cancers combined. In the United Kingdom, there are more than 250,000 episodes of sepsis annually, with at least 44,000 people dying as a result (UK Sepsis Trust, 2017).

In the same way that healthcare practitioners are encouraged to think 'could this chest pain be cardiac in origin?', NICE (2016, updated 2017) guidance encourages healthcare practitioners to consider 'Could this be sepsis?' with anyone presenting with a possible infection.

A summary of Mary's initial observations on admission to the emergency department are presented in Box 7.4.

Box 7.4 Mary's initial observations

Miss Mary Norton is a 49 year old lady who is usually fit and well. She was admitted to the emergency department complaining of pain and tenderness within her right upper limb. She thinks that she scratched her right index finger whilst gardening but is unable to remember this clearly. She has developed defuse inflammation and reduced movement in her right hand and pain in the right axilla. Her friend has accompanied her to the emergency department. Mary weighs 75 kgs.

Airway

- Mary is able to speak in full sentences

(Continued)

Breathing

- Respiratory rate: 30 breaths per minute (bpm)
- Oxygen saturation levels: 92% on air
- Chest clear on examination

Circulation

- Blood pressure: 90/40 mmHg
- Heart rate: 115 beats per minute, Sinus Tachycardia
- Temperature: 37.8°C
- Urine output unknown
- Capillary refill time (CRT): 2 seconds

Disability

- New onset confusion on ACVPU, disorientated and unable to clearly recall history
- Pain score 2/3 (difficult to accurately record due to confusion), complaining of right upper limb pain
- Blood glucose: 7.0 mmol/l

Exposure

- Pressure areas intact
- Diffuse inflammation in the right hand extending from finger to her axilla

Management of sepsis

Management of sepsis in the UK is guided and operationalised by three key sources: the NICE NG51 *Sepsis: Recognition, diagnosis and early management guideline* (NICE, 2016a, updated 2017), the Third international consensus definitions for sepsis and septic shock (sepsis-3) (Singer et al., 2016) and *The Sepsis Manual* (UK Sepsis Trust, 2017). Sepsis is a time critical condition; the UK Sepsis Trust's (2017) focus on early recognition and urgent intervention identifying that for every hour that appropriate antibiotic is delayed, there is an 8% increase in mortality.

Assessment

Following on from the initial set of observations that were carried out, a National Early Warning Score (2) (Royal College of Physicians [RCP], 2017) was calculated for Mary. This found Mary had a high NEWS2 score of 13, which necessitated immediate referral to a specialist registrar and emergency response team such as the critical care outreach team (RCP, 2017). This was because Mary was at risk of rapid deterioration and death as confirmed by the score of 3 using Quick Sequential Organ Failure Assessment (SOFA) (Singer et al., 2016). See Table 7.1 for Quick SOFA criteria.

Table 7.1   Quick SOFA criteria

qSOFA criteria The score is calculated by giving 1 point for each of the following prognostic features:	Mary's score
Respiratory rate ≥ 22/min	1
Altered mentation	1
Systolic blood pressure ≤ 100mmHg	1
Total	3/3

The nurse established from Mary's accompanying friend that the confusion Mary was presenting with was new and totally out of character for her and in line with NICE (2016a, updated 2017) guidance temperature should not be used as the sole predictor of sepsis.

In line with the National Confidential Enquiry into patient outcome and death (NCEPOD) report *Just say sepsis!* (NCEPOD, 2015), the nurse understood to implement the Sepsis Six bundle immediately.

The Sepsis Six bundle involved:

1. Commencing oxygen therapy for Mary through a non-rebreathe oxygen mask at 15l/min with the aim of keeping her SpO_2 above 94% (NICE, 2016a, updated 2017).
2. Taking blood cultures to identify the type of bacteria.
3. Administering intravenous broad spectrum antibiotics at maximum recommended dose (NICE, 2016a, updated 2017).
4. Measuring Mary's serum lactate, if it was above 4 mmol/l – referral to critical care outreach had already been implemented on the basis of her high NEWS2.
5. Administering IV fluids (crystalloids). Mary had a fluid bolus of 500 mls of crystalloid over 15 minutes (NICE, 2013, updated May 2017). The fluid continued not exceeding 30 mls/kg.
6. Inserting a urinary catheter and measuring Mary's hourly urine output, which should be at 0.5ml/kg/hour which in Mary's case is 38 mls/hr.

Whilst this was being administered within 1 hour of admission to the emergency department (UK Sepsis Trust, 2017; NICE, 2016a, updated 2017), Mary's mental state was monitored using ACVPU and urinalysis and a chest X-ray were performed. A thorough clinical examination to look for sources of infection was undertaken. Mary's pain in her right arm was also assessed and an opioid analgesic administered; paracetamol was administered intravenously in light of the mild temperature rise. The area of inflammation was marked on her arm to enable any spread to be identified and her arm carefully inspected for any breaks in the skin. The nurse recognised that Mary was at high risk of tissue breakdown in light of her impaired circulation and infection. Cellulitis was suspected as the source of infection. Cellulitis is a spreading bacterial infection of the dermis and subcutaneous tissues.

NICE (2016a) also identify that in addition to the steps of the Sepsis Six, venous blood testing should include:

- Venous blood gas including glucose
- Full blood count
- C-reactive protein
- Urea and electrolytes
- Creatinine
- Clotting screen

Based on Mary's high NEWS2 and qSOFA score, a decision was made to admit Mary to the high dependency unit where she could be closely observed. In line with NICE (2016a, updated 2017) guidance, the nurse facilitated Mary's friend to contact her family and on their arrival explained to Mary and to them that Mary had sepsis, the investigations that had been undertaken and what the management plan was. She was careful to communicate with them clearly, not using medical jargon and gave them time to ask questions.

Ongoing management

Development of sepsis has led to decreased tissue perfusion and Mary is at risk of septic shock if this is not corrected. Widespread capillary leakage and mal-distribution of blood volume between the three fluid compartments (intracellular, intravascular and the interstitial) has caused swelling and a relative hypovolaemia, which will cause further hypoperfusion and pain due to pressure on nerve endings. The kidneys are receiving less blood volume and compensatory mechanisms are failing. Inflammation and heat throughout Mary's right arm are evidence of vessel vasodilation in response to the bacterial invasion and the release of a large amount of cytokines (inflammatory markers) support this. Mary's blood results indicate C-reactive protein (CRP) >285 mg/l and a White Cell Count (WBC) 18,000/mm3, both of which are elevated. Mary is also at risk of AKI development due to pre-renal factors (volume depletion) or intra-renal factors such as inflammatory markers could produce direct damage to kidney tissues and other organs.

To manage this situation, Mary was commenced on specific antibiotics on receipt of the blood culture results. Intravenous fluid administration was reassessed after the initial bolus and a further 500ml crystalloid administered.

Mary's observations on admission to the high dependency unit following commencement of the Sepsis Six are shown in Box 7.5.

Box 7.5 Observations on admission to the high dependency unit

Airway

- Mary is able to speak in full sentences

Breathing

- Respiratory rate: 20 breaths per minute (bpm)
- Oxygen saturation levels: 97% on 15l oxygen
- Chest clear on examination

Circulation

- Blood pressure: 100/55 mmHg
- Heart rate: 110 beats per minute, Sinus Tachycardia
- Temperature: 37.5°C
- Urine output: 38ml/h
- Capillary refill time (CRT): 2 seconds

Disability

- Alert on ACVPU
- Pain score 1/3 complaining of right upper limb tenderness
- Blood glucose: 7.0 mmol/l

Exposure

- Pressure areas intact
- Diffuse inflammation in the right hand extending from finger to her axilla

---

Management on the HDU

Airway and breathing

Mary's airway patency presents no concern on admission to HDU. Her oxygen perfusion has improved with administration of high flow oxygen and is within the target 94–98% (BTS, 2017) and this can now be titrated down, switching from the non-rebreathe mask to a venturi device. Mary's SpO$_2$ should be carefully monitored for five minutes after each change in oxygen delivery. Mary's respiratory rate has reduced in keeping with her improved oxygen perfusion.

Circulation

Mary needs to receive fluid therapy to ensure her blood pressure and cardiac output remain acceptable and a strict fluid balance record made. Heart rate should be monitored, expecting that this will decrease as the inflammatory response decreases. The administration of the antibiotics will treat the underlying cause, which is the cellulitis. This should eventually reduce the capillary permeability as the infection recedes. Urine output needs to be monitored hourly to ensure Mary does not develop an AKI and the catheter removed at the first opportunity when Mary's cardiovascular status is stable. Her temperature needs to be taken and the capillary refill time monitored as an indication of peripheral tissue perfusion.

Disability

ACVPU needs to be undertaken with the NEWS2 scoring. This will demonstrate how effective Mary's cerebral perfusion is and is particularly key in light of her earlier confusion as an indicator of likely sepsis. Blood glucose levels need to be monitored to evaluate the sympathetic nervous system (SNS) response to this acute illness – Mary's glucose of 7.0 mmol/l is within an acceptable parameter. Mary will continue to need assessment of her pain within her right arm and appropriate analgesia administered. Assessment should utilise a pain scoring tool such as a numerical score 0–3, which equates to the WHO analgesic ladder, alongside a more comprehensive assessment that considers the nature, location and aggravating factors (see Chapter 9 for discussion of acute pain assessment tools).

Exposure

Mary's pressure areas and particularly the fragile skin around the inflamed area on her right arm need to be monitored regularly, a minimum of two hourly. Mary is at high risk of experiencing tissue breakdown and worsening the development of sepsis. Mary should be encouraged to mobilise early to offset this risk.

Monitoring using the NEWS2 should continue regularly until Mary has responded to treatment and is safe to discharge. On discharge it is important that the team looking after Mary explain to her and her family what sepsis is, the tests and investigations that have been done, give her instruction on which symptoms to monitor such as the currently receding inflammation and tenderness to her right arm, when and how to get medical attention if it is needed urgently (NICE, 2016a, updated 2017). The discharging team need to ensure continuity of care for Mary by informing her GP of her admission and diagnosis and arranging follow up. There is good evidence of the potential psychological and physical long term effects of sepsis referred to as 'post sepsis syndrome' thought to be due to the changes in the microcirculation and the action of pro-inflammatory cytokines (UK Sepsis Trust, 2017). Therefore it is important that Mary is aware of national charities and support groups that may offer ongoing help as she comes to terms with her diagnosis.

Conclusion

A case study considering a patient, Mary Norton, presenting with sepsis has been considered, outlining the relevant pathophysiology and incorporating evidence-based interventions and management strategies.

CASE STUDY 7.3: HYPOVOLAEMIA – SARA ELSON

The third case study in this chapter focuses on the most common type of circulatory collapse – hypovolaemic shock. The task force for the European Intensive Care Society state 'shock is best defined as a life-threatening, generalized form of acute circulatory failure associated with inadequate oxygen utilization by the cells. It is a state in which circulation is unable to deliver sufficient oxygen to meet the demands of the tissues, resulting in cellular dysfunction' (Cecconi et al., 2014).

Although the causes of shock and patient presentation are variable as identified in the previous chapter and within the first case study, the end result of cellular hypoxia is the same and this may be life threatening.

Three stages of shock are commonly recognised in text books with an initial phase preceding these where overt signs and symptoms are less obvious. This initial response in shock is dependent on the person's age and previous health state. Stages of shock comprise continuous and complex processes and there is usually no sudden transition from one stage to another.

Stages of shock:

- Initial
- Compensatory/reversible
- Progressive/decompensated
- Refractory/irreversible

Initial stage of shock

During the initial phase of shock, cellular change is occurring. When cells are deprived of oxygen due to the reduction in blood volume, the mitochondria can no longer continue to produce adenosine triphosphate (ATP), which is essential for the generation of energy in the cells. Without oxygen, the cells start to function anaerobically, which is much less efficient. The by-products lactic and pyruvic acid cause the body to develop a systemic metabolic acidosis. This is harmful to the cells and needs to be removed by the blood and broken down in the liver; however this process also requires oxygen.

Activity 7.2

What change in a person's vital signs might be seen during the initial phase of shock?

Compensatory stage of shock

If the underlying cause of the reduced tissue perfusion is not corrected, this will initiate a series of compensatory mechanisms referred to as the compensatory stage of shock. Some texts refer to this as the 'reversible' stage of shock, which is a key concept. Timely and appropriate assessment and intervention at this point can reduce morbidity and mortality. In the early stages of compensatory shock where blood pressure cannot adequately perfuse the body with oxygen and nutrients, a series of neural, hormonal and chemical compensatory mechanisms are initiated in an attempt to restore homeostasis and maintain blood flow to the vital organs (Migliozzi, 2017).

Neural compensation – the sympathetic nervous system regulates blood flow and pressure through its ability to increase heart rate and total peripheral resistance. Baroreceptors and chemoreceptors located in the carotid sinus and aortic arch detect the reduction in blood pressure and relay messages to the vasomotor centre in the medulla oblongata.

Hormonal compensation – initiated by the activation of the sympathetic nervous system, the decrease in renal blood flow initiates the action of the renin-angiotensin-aldosterone system (RAAS). The renal medulla secretes adrenaline and noradrenaline, which increases heart rate and causes the coronary arteries to dilate, increasing blood flow to the heart to meet the oxygen demand. Fluid loss is reduced due to the increased amount of anti-diuretic hormone released from the anterior pituitary gland and the anti-natriuretic properties of aldosterone.

Chemical compensation – a reduction in cardiac output leads to a decrease in blood flow to the lungs detected by peripheral and central chemoreceptors. This results in an increased rate of ventilation. However this hyperventilation causes a reduction in carbon dioxide, which impacts on blood flow and perfusion to the brain potentially causing restlessness and confusion (Migliozzi, 2017).

If the compensatory mechanisms fail to restore blood pressure and tissue perfusion and the underlying cause of the circulatory failure has not been addressed, Sara will progress to the next stage of shock.

Progressive stage of shock

The progressive stage of shock occurs when the initial compensatory mechanisms fail to restore an adequate blood pressure and tissue perfusion. Timely and appropriate recognition and intervention in the early stages of this decompensated stage can save the person's life. If the underlying problem is not recognised, for example an internal haemorrhage, tissue perfusion will be impaired and tissue damage will occur. Vasoconstriction continues to occur, shunting blood from the peripheries to the vital organs, but this is at the expense of the microcirculation resulting in ischaemia at the extremities. Impaired cellular metabolism occurs as a result of an inadequate blood supply of oxygen and nutrients, and decreased levels of oxygen cause the cells to switch from aerobic metabolism to anaerobic metabolism leading to acidosis. Prolonged anaerobic metabolism results in a reduction in the production of the body fuel adenotriphosphate (ATP), which leads to a failure of the sodium potassium pump situated on the cell membrane. Its usual action in restoring homeostatic balance in the cell is impaired and cellular wall permeability is increased, resulting in sodium ions accumulating within the cell causing swelling and a deterioration in function. Peripheral vascular resistance is further decreased by release of bradykinin and histamine, both of which have vasodilating properties and impair venous return. This further decreases blood pressure and cardiac output leading to cellular hypoxia.

Hypoxia impairs cerebral function and can lead to confusion, restlessness and impair conscious level. As impairment of the microcirculation proceeds in the progressive stage, thrombosis and ischaemia of organs such as the bowel and pancreas become common.

Refractory stage of shock

At this stage, the vital organs have failed and the effects of shock can no longer be reversed. The continued decrease in cardiac output means the body is unable to respond to any form of intervention and multiple organ system failure occurs; death will occur within a few hours.

A summary of Sara's initial observations are presented in Box 7.6.

Box 7.6 Sara's initial observations

Sara Elson is a 22 year old store assistant who was thrown from her bicycle and injured in a road traffic collision. She has been admitted to the ward with abdominal pain and large bruises along the left side of her body. Over the past 12 hours she reported that she was feeling increasingly unwell with raised intensity of pain. Sara does not have significant past medical or surgical history but she is becoming more hypotensive and tachycardic. Sara weighs 57 kgs.

Airway

- Sara is able to speak one or two words

Breathing

- Respiratory rate: 27 breaths per minute (bpm)
- Oxygen saturation levels: 83% on 3L oxygen per minute
- Chest clear on examination

Circulation

- Blood pressure: 84/52 mmHg
- Heart rate: 127 beats per minute, Sinus Tachycardia
- Temperature: 36°C
- Urine output last 3 hours: 30 mls, 20 mls and 20 mls
- Capillary refill time (CRT): 4 seconds

Disability

- Alert on ACVPU, but distressed and anxious
- Pain score 2/3; complaining of moderate abdominal pain not localising and is dull in nature
- Blood glucose: 8.0 mmol/l

Exposure

- Pressure areas intact
- Skin and mouth are dry

Management of hypovolaemia

Management of hypovolaemia in the UK is guided by early recognition of the signs of shock utilising an early warning score NEWS2 (RCP, 2017) and treating the underlying cause of the circulatory failure, which frequently focuses on fluid resuscitation in line with NICE CG174 *Intravenous fluid therapy in adults in hospital* (NICE, 2013, updated May 2017).

The NICE intravenous fluid therapy guideline (NICE, 2013, updated May 2017) was a long awaited guideline that aimed to address the prescribing errors, lack of knowledge of fluid and electrolyte needs and fluid composition that were identified in practice. A National Confidential Enquiry into Patient Outcomes and Death (NCEPOD) in 1999 identified that a significant number of patients were dying as a result of being given too much or too little fluid with some complications potentially being fatal. Out of this came an emphasis on pre-scription of intravenous fluids and focus on improving the standard of monitoring and record keeping. A more recent report, albeit focusing on acute pancreatitis, *Treat the cause* (NCEPOD, 2016), continued to identify that intravenous fluid management was 'inadequate' in a signifi-cant percentage of patients.

Assessment

Following on from the initial set of observations that were carried out, a National Early Warning Score (2) (Royal College of Physicians [RCP], 2017) was calculated for Sara. This found Sara had a high NEWS2 score of 14, which necessitated immediate referral to a specialist registrar and emergency response team such as the critical care outreach team (RCP, 2017).

Whilst the admitting nurse was contacting the emergency response team, she asked another nurse to ensure that Sara had a patent intravenous cannula in place and to increase the oxygen concentration delivery in line with the British Thoracic Society guidelines for emergency oxygen use (2017). The nurse had a high suspicion that Sara had signs of hypovolaemic shock due to haemorrhaging internally as indicated by the bruising to her left side and abdominal pain, and required emergency fluid resuscitation in line with Algorithm 1 and 2 of the NICE (2013, updated May 2017) guidelines.

Algorithm 1 indicates that a patient may need fluid resuscitation (NICE, 2013, updated May 2017) if:

- Systolic BP <100 mmHg
- Heart rate >90 bpm
- Capillary refill >2 s or peripheries cold to touch
- Respiratory rate >20 breaths per min
- NEWS ≥ 5
- 45° leg raising suggest fluid responsiveness

Activity 7.3

Passive leg raising (PLR) is a test that predicts whether cardiac output will increase with volume expansion. No fluid is infused, PLR mimics a fluid challenge in transferring lower body fluid to the right side of the heart. Conduct a literature search to review the reliability of this test.

Assessment by the emergency response team and specialist registrar confirmed that Sara is hypovolaemic and met these indications therefore Algorithm 2 Fluid Resuscitation was implemented. Sara was moving from the compensatory stage of shock to the progressive stage and required immediate intervention to identify the underlying cause and intervention to improve tissue perfusion. In line with NICE (2013, updated May 2017) guidelines, a Crystalloid bolus 500 mls (containing sodium in the range of 130–154 mmol/l over less than 15 minutes) was administered.

Algorithm 2 also emphasises identifying the cause of the deficit and responding appropriately. Therefore the specialist registrar requested an urgent CT scan with a view to detecting any internal haemorrhage and need for emergency surgery to stem the bleeding.

Reassessment is a key part of fluid resuscitation and whilst the internal haemorrhage was confirmed and preparation for theatre made, Sara was reassessed using an ABCDE approach and received further boluses of 500ml Crystalloid administered according to her response.

Likely fluid and electrolyte needs were assessed in line with NICE (2013, updated May 2017) guidelines, taking into account:

- Sara's history – oral intake had been limited to sips of water since admission. Sara reported feeling thirsty, urine output was decreasing over the last three hours since admission. There were no underlying comorbidities.
- In addition to pulse, blood pressure and capillary refill already measured, assessment of JVP and presence of oedema were assessed for.

Oedema is the excessive accumulation of interstitial fluid where fluid is forced out of the blood vessels. Oedema may occur from leakage at the vessel site, i.e. cannulation puncture, increased capillary permeability, decreased concentration of plasma proteins (low plasma oncotic pressure), cell membrane damage or due to increased extracellular fluid. If the left side of the heart is overloaded, fluid will back up in lungs (pulmonary oedema), when the right side is overloaded, fluid backs up in the body. Sara had no clinical signs of oedema being present. Sara had no observable signs of oedema developing.

Jugular Venous Pressure (JVP) is the indirectly observed pressure of the internal jugular vein. This becomes elevated when there is an imbalance of blood flow into and out of the right heart either due to increased blood flow or increased resistance to right heart ejection (Ward, 2014).

A further measure of tissue perfusion recommended by NICE's major trauma guidelines (NICE, 2016b) is measurement of lactate as this may be a more responsive indicator of shock due to the late changes that occur in measurement of blood pressure. Lactate is the by-product of cells functioning anaerobically and measured clinically by arterial blood gas measurement (ABG). Sara had an ABG sample taken when she was on the ward receiving 15l/min oxygen therapy. The results are presented in Box 7.7.

Box 7.7 Sara's arterial blood gas result

pH 7.30 mmol

PaO_2 9.2 kPa

$PaCO_2$ 4.2 kPa

HCO_3 18 mmol/l

Lactate 4.0 mmol/l

Base excess –9

The ABG was analysed using the five-step approach as presented in Chapter 4. Sara has evidence of a metabolic acidosis indicated by the reduced pH and bicarbonate. Oxygenation on 15l oxygen therapy was seen as acceptable. The lactate is high, demonstrating reduced tissue perfusion and the presence of anaerobic respiration due to the development of hypovolaemic shock. The elevated lactate is further confirmation of the need to fluid resuscitate Sara.

The nurse commenced a fluid balance monitoring chart to accurately record input and output in line with NICE (2013, updated May 2017) guidance. Recording of fluid balance has been identified over many years as notoriously inadequate with many healthcare staff familiar with abbreviations such as OTT ('out to toilet') and incomplete charts. More influentially, the Report of the Mid Staffordshire NHS Foundation Public Inquiry (Francis, 2013) found there was poor practice in relation to recording fluid balance. Sara's nurse was aware that the NMC (2015, updated 2018) also emphasise the importance of accurate and timely record keeping.

In line with NICE (2013, updated May 2017) guidelines, laboratory assessment of full blood count (FBC), urea, creatinine and electrolytes were requested along with cross matching for blood compatibility.

The treatment goal here is the preservation and improvement of Sara's tissue perfusion. This is dependent on adequate supply and transport of oxygen, as well as the cellular ability to use it. Achieving the appropriate haemoglobin and cardiac output is essential for the transport of oxygen. Fluid therapy aims to optimise preload by increasing intravascular volume, improving cardiac performance to improve cardiac output.

Types of fluids: Tonicity

Fluid can be divided into three different types according to its tonicity:

- Isotonic
- Hypotonic
- Hypertonic

Tonicity refers to the concentration of ions in the fluid and understanding some of this chemistry will aid understanding of the choice of intravenous fluid for resuscitation and maintenance fluids.

Isotonic fluid has the same solute concentration as another solution therefore there is no net fluid shift. *Hypotonic* solutions have a lower concentration whereas *hypertonic* solutions have a higher concentration. Table 7.2 gives some simple common examples of tonicity of fluids.

Table 7.2   Tonicity of fluids

Hypotonic	Isotonic	Hypertonic
0.45% sodium chloride	0.9% sodium chloride	Semi synthetic starch, e.g. Gelofusine
0.18% sodium chloride	Hartmann's solution	(Albumin)
	(5% glucose)	

Isotonic solutions given intravenously do not result in any significant fluid shift across cellular or vascular membranes. Isotonic fluids follow the normal principles of fluid movement within the body, filtering out at the arterial end of the capillary and being reabsorbed at the venous end. A *hypertonic* solution given intravenously will draw fluids from the cells and interstitial spaces into the vasculature. A *hypotonic* solution given intravenously will cause fluids to leave the vasculature for the interstitial and intracellular spaces.

Activity 7.4

Before you read any further, reflect on the fluids you have seen administered in practice. Can you identify why they were chosen and the effect on fluid distribution they would have?

Types of resuscitation fluid

There are two types of resuscitation fluids: crystalloids and colloids.

Crystalloids – crystalloid solutions contain small molecules and flow easily from the vasculature to the cells and tissues. They can be isotonic, hypotonic or hypertonic. There is an increasing recommendation for the use of Hartmann's solution, particularly for post-operative surgical patients. Hartmann's is isotonic with blood; this means it contains normal physiological (serum) electrolyte levels diluted in water (sodium, chloride, lactate, potassium and calcium). The advantage of this is that this type of fluid can fill the three fluid compartments. Initially it should fill the intravascular compartment, increasing the circulatory volume and perfusion pressure (blood pressure) before perfusing the intracellular and interstitial space. 0.9% sodium chloride (NaCl) shares the same advantages as Hartmann's solution, however despite being referred to as 'normal', the solution is not physiologically normal because it has a higher concentration of chloride ions than plasma. This high load of chlorine can cause a hyperchloraemic metabolic acidosis. 5% Glucose does not stay in the intravascular compartment as it has a low osmotic pressure. It is therefore not used to increase perfusion pressure or for resuscitation. It is used to re-hydrate the intracellular compartment as fluid will have moved from this compartment to the intravascular compartment as part of the compensatory mechanisms taking place.

Activity 7.5

Access the NICE resource for composition of crystalloids to compare them to plasma: www.nice.org.uk/guidance/cg174/resources/composition-of-commonly-used-crystalloids-table-pdf-191662813

Colloids – stay in the intravascular compartment longer as they are made up of weightier proteins that exert an increased osmotic pull; they are all hypertonic. Optimising the osmotic pressure will attract and retain fluid in the vasculature meaning lower volumes of colloid fluid are required for a comparable result to crystalloids. However, their increased risk of allergic reactions over crystalloids is weighed up in their use. Albumin is not advised for use in general resuscitation but may be used in sepsis. Human albumin is the magnetic force responsible for driving oncotic pressure and can be an effective treatment option in the context of the mal-distribution of blood volume due to capillary leakage.

A systematic review by Lewis et al. (2018) concluded that using colloids compared to crystalloids for fluid replacement probably makes little or no difference to the number of critically ill people who die. In line with NICE fluid resuscitation guidance (NICE, 2013, updated May 2017), Sara received crystalloid fluids.

Blood products

As part of Sara's blood profile, samples will be taken for a full blood count (FBC) to determine haemoglobin level (Hb) and group and cross matching. Part of Sara's fluid resuscitation may include the administration of blood products in order to ensure sufficient oxygen carrying capacity to the vital organs and replace blood loss from the intravascular space. Prothrombin time (PT) and Activated Partial Thromboplastin time (APTT) will be measured to assess for any deranged clotting.

Administration of blood products is a high risk procedure and there are well established clinical protocols in every clinical area to reduce risk and preserve patient safety.

Time out: Review the transfusion guidelines in your clinical area. What is the bedside check? Do you know what the potential adverse effects of transfusion are?

Review the guidance here for further information: www.transfusionguidelines.org/transfusion-handbook; and Serious Hazards of Transfusion annual reports here: www.shotuk.org/shot-reports/

NICE blood transfusion guidance NG24 (NICE, 2015) considers a transfusion threshold of 70 g/litre Hb for patients who do not have major haemorrhage, acute coronary syndrome or chronic anaemia. Administration of platelets, fresh frozen plasma and Cryoprecipitate may be indicated for patients who are actively bleeding and have abnormal coagulation tests.

Emergency surgery was carried out on Sara to remove a ruptured spleen and stem the active bleeding. In theatre she received two units of compatible blood and further crystalloid to stabilise her blood pressure. Routine maintenance fluids to meet normal daily electrolyte requirements of 25–30 mmol/l /day and 1 mmol/kg/day of sodium, potassium and chloride water were commenced. She had been catheterised and a urometer was in situ. Analgesia had been administered prior to surgery and in theatre (see Chapter 9 on acute pain management). For monitoring and continued stabilisation of her care, it was agreed that Sara be admitted to the high dependency unit (HDU). Sara's observations on admission to HDU are detailed in Box 7.8.

Box 7.8 Sara's observations on admission to HDU

Airway

- Sara is sleepy following surgery but is able to speak in short sentences

(Continued)

Breathing

- Respiratory rate: 14 breaths per minute (bpm)
- Oxygen saturation levels: 97%
- Chest clear on examination

Circulation

- Blood pressure: 110/60 mmHg
- Heart rate: 82 beats per minute, Sinus rhythm
- Temperature: 36.5°C
- Urine output: 35 ml/h
- Capillary refill time (CRT): 1 second

Disability

- Alert on ACVPU
- Pain score 1/3, some guarding of surgical site and abdomen
- Blood glucose: 6.5 mmol/l

Exposure

- Pressure areas intact
- Skin and mouth are dry

Management on the HDU

Airway and breathing

Sara's airway patency presents no concern on admission to HDU. Her oxygen perfusion has improved with administration of high flow oxygen and is within the target 94–98% (BTS, 2017) and has now been titrated down until the supplementary oxygen has been removed. Sara's SpO_2 will be carefully monitored to ensure that she maintains this level of oxygen perfusion. Sara's respiratory rate has reduced in keeping with her improved oxygen perfusion circulatory volume. Sara will benefit from physiotherapy input to aid the lungs' recovery after the general anaesthetic.

Circulation

Sara needs to receive fluid therapy to ensure her blood pressure and cardiac output remain acceptable and a strict fluid balance record made. As soon as is possible she should be encouraged to eat and drink normally. Her lactate measurement should be repeated as an indicator that tissue perfusion has improved along with regular monitoring of her urea and electrolyte balance. Urine output needs to be monitored hourly to ensure Sara does not develop an AKI and the catheter removed at the first opportunity when Sara's cardiovascular status is stable. Current output meets the threshold of 0.5ml/kg/hour. Repeat FBC will need to be taken to detect potential anaemia and WBC count reviewed following splenectomy. Prophylactic antibiotics should be administered following surgery and the qSOFA criteria observed as indicators of sepsis. Low dose antibiotics will need to be continued for life to prevent bacterial infections as the spleen has been removed. Temperature needs to be taken and the capillary refill time monitored as an indication of peripheral tissue perfusion.

Disability

ACVPU needs to be undertaken with the NEWS2 scoring. This will demonstrate how effective Sara's cerebral perfusion is. Blood glucose levels need to be monitored to evaluate the sympathetic nervous system (SNS) response to this acute illness. Sara's glucose of 6.5 mmol/l is within an acceptable parameter. Sara will continue to need assessment of her post-operative pain and appropriate analgesia administered. Non-pharmacological options such as support of the bruised area with a rolled up towel on movement could also be employed. Assessment should utilise a pain scoring tool such as a numerical score 0–3, which equates to the WHO analgesic ladder, alongside a more comprehensive assessment that considers the nature, location and aggravating factors (see Chapter 9 for discussion of acute pain assessment and management).

Exposure

Sara's pressure areas need to be monitored regularly, a minimum of two hourly. Sara is at high risk of experiencing tissue breakdown due to the episode of acute illness. Sara should be encouraged to mobilise early to offset this risk.

Monitoring using the NEWS2 should continue regularly until Sara has responded to treatment and is safe to discharge. During the monitoring and stabilisation phase it is key that Sara's psychological, social and spiritual needs are also met. As a 22 year old young woman experiencing a traumatic injury she will feel distressed and anxious about the hospital admission, interventions and the future.

On discharge it is important that the team looking after Sara explain to her and her family the implications of spleen removal, the tests and investigations that have been done, give her instruction on which symptoms to monitor such as signs of infection. It would be advisable for

Sara to carry or wear some medical ID and to make sure that she remains up-to-date with vaccinations as the spleen's function in immunity has been removed. The discharging team need to ensure continuity of care for Sara by informing her GP of her admission and diagnosis and arranging follow up. Therefore it is important that Sara is aware of national charities and support groups that may offer ongoing help as she comes to terms with her diagnosis.

Conclusion

A case study considering a patient, Sara Elson presenting with hypovolaemic shock has been considered, outlining the relevant pathophysiology and incorporating evidence-based interventions and management strategies.

CASE STUDY 7.4: AKI – RONALD HUNT

The fourth case study in this chapter looks at a patient who has developed AKI.

> Acute kidney injury, previously known as acute renal failure, encompasses a wide spectrum of injury to the kidneys, not just kidney failure (NICE, 2019).

AKI is characterised by a rapid reduction in kidney function that can result in organ failure and the need for renal replacement therapy. Pathophysiology and diagnostic criteria for AKI have been presented in Chapter 6, focusing on monitoring creatinine levels with or without urine output. AKI occurs as a result of volume depletion and hypoperfusion to the kidneys, decreased renal blood flow and/or toxic inflammatory injury to the kidneys (Tait & Hanson, 2016). There has been a particular emphasis for healthcare practitioners to 'Think Kidneys' as AKI is seen in 13–18% of all people admitted to hospital, with older adults being particularly affected (NICE, 2019). The NCEPOD report (2009) *Adding insult to injury*, identified that only 50% of AKI care was of good quality; its recommendations for future practice have been incorporated into clinical guidance (NICE, 2019).

Key to improving the care and treatment of people with AKI is identifying those who are most at risk. Box 7.9 identifies who is most at risk according to NICE (2019).

Box 7.9 Identifying AKI in patients

- Acute illness and/or deteriorating NEWS2 score
- Long term conditions such as chronic kidney disease, liver failure, heart failure, diabetes
- Oliguria (urine output <0.5ml/kg/hour)

(Continued)

- Hypovolaemia
- Age ≥ 65 years
- Neurological/cognitive impairment limiting ready access to fluids
- Use of drugs with nephrotoxic potential (such as NSAIDs, aminoglycosides, angiotensin-converting enzyme [ACE] inhibitors, angiotensin II receptor antagonists [ARBs] and diuretics) in last week
- Use of iodinated contrast agents in last week
- Urological obstruction
- Sepsis

A summary of Ronald's observations on calling the nurse to say he was feeling very unwell are presented in Box 7.10

Box 7.10 Ronald's initial observations

Ronald Hunt is a 75 year old gentleman who had a hernia repair five days ago. Over the last 24 hours he reported that he was increasingly feeling unwell. He has a four-day history of nausea and vomiting, and is now unable to take oral fluids. His past medical history includes increasingly debilitating rheumatoid arthritis, which has been treated with non-steroidal anti-inflammatory drugs (NSAIDS). Over the last 12 hours he has had six episodes of diarrhoea and vomited approximately 500 mls. Ronald weighed 75 kgs at his pre-operation check.

Airway

- Ronald is able to speak in full sentences

Breathing

- Respiratory rate: 20 breaths per minute (bpm)
- Oxygen saturation levels: 95% on air
- Chest clear on examination

Circulation

- Blood pressure: 100/70 mmHg
- Heart rate: 95 beats per minute, Sinus Tachycardia
- Temperature: 36.8°C
- Urine output last 3 hours: 60 mls, 20 mls, 0 mls

(Continued)

- Urea: 17 mmol/l
- Creatinine: 258 µmol/l
- Potassium: 6.7 mmol/l

Disability

- Alert on ACVPU, orientated to place and time but distressed
- Pain score 1/3, complaining of mild abdominal pain
- Blood glucose: 8.0 mmol/l

Exposure

- Pressure areas intact
- Skin dry with reduced turgor

Management of AKI in the UK is guided by early recognition of the signs of AKI in order to prevent deterioration and loss of renal function. Key clinical guidance from NICE NG148 (2019) *Acute kidney injury: prevention, detection and management*. Use of the RIFLE, AKIN or KDIGO (see Chapter 6) criteria are recommended for staging the grade of injury.

Assessment

Following on from the initial set of observations that were carried out, a NEWS2 (Royal College of Physicians [RCP], 2017) was calculated for Ronald. This found Ronald had a NEWS2 score of 4. A minimum of four to six hourly monitoring is recommended by the RCP (2017) at this level; however the nurse caring for Ronald was concerned that his urine output had deteriorated in the last couple of hours and he had reported several episodes of diarrhoea and had vomited. She gathered his observation and fluid balance chart together and looked up his blood results in preparation for making a SBAR call. Her SBAR call is recorded in Box 7.11.

Box 7.11 SBAR call to the surgical team caring for Ronald

Situation, Background, Assessment, Recommendation (SBAR) (NHS Improvement, 2018)

S: I am Alice, a registered nurse on Ward B. I am calling about Ronald Hunt. I am calling because I am concerned that Ronald feels increasingly unwell, his respiratory rate is 20 bpm,

(Continued)

oxygen saturation 95% on air, his blood pressure is 100/70 mmHg, his heart rate is 95 bpm. His urine output is decreasing and he has not passed urine in the last hour. His creatinine is 258 μmol/l, his urea is 17 mmol/l and his potassium is 6.7 mmol/l. He also has diarrhoea and has vomited. His NEWS2 is 4.

B: Ronald had a hernia repair five days ago and has been slow to recover. He has a history of rheumatoid arthritis.

A: I'm not sure what the problem is but I am concerned that Ronald is dehydrated and not passing urine.

R: I need you to come and see the patient urgently. Would you like me to arrange anything in the meantime?

Initial assessment of Ronald identified that he met several of the risk factors for development of AKI: he was over 65 years of age, had a deteriorating NEWS2 score, was oliguric and was receiving a NSAID for treatment of rheumatoid arthritis.

The clinical course of AKI can be divided into four phases:

- Initiating – occurs when the kidneys are injured and is caused by any trigger that reduces tissue perfusion or causes toxic renal damage. It can last from hours to days.
- Oliguric (maintenance) – this can last from 5 days to over 15 days. Over time endocrine problems such as reduced erythropoietin production, decreased tubular transport, reduced urine formation and lowered glomerular filtration occur. Renal healing will begin to occur, with the basement membrane being replaced with fibrous scar tissue and the nephron clogged with inflammatory products (Davies, 2013). The patient is particularly susceptible to bleeding and infection during this stage.
- Diuretic – as the kidney heals it begins to regain its lost function, depending on the severity of the injury. Urine output increases to normal levels of up to three litres per day (Davies, 2013).
- Recovery – normal renal function becomes established; however this can take from several months to over a year. It may take some time for the renal tubules to filter, reabsorb and secrete adequately.

So, let us apply this to Ronald's case. Assessment by the surgical team confirms that Ronald is at risk of AKI with an elevated creatinine level of 258 μmol/l confirming that injury to the kidney was taking place. Urine output has decreased over the last two hours placing him in the oliguric phase, along with signs of dehydration due to the diarrhoea and vomiting.

Presence of a nephrotoxic agent (NSAID) poses risk of intra-renal injury whilst the dehydration indicates a hypovolaemic picture posing a pre-renal injury threat. Whilst pathophysiology surrounding intra-renal damage is complex, it is understood that an interruption to the blood supply causes renal ischaemia. The depth of this damage seems to be variable in different patient groups.

The longer the damage persists the greater the risk of necrosis developing. Debris from red blood cells, damaged cells and cellular debris will build up in the tissue and prevent the flow of filtrate through the glomerulus. Ischaemic damage to the epithelial cells reduces their permeability and damage to the capillary endothelium allows fluid to seep from the capillaries into the tissues and cause cellular swelling and tubular obstruction. Ischaemic damage results in deep lesions to the tubular epithelium and basement membrane – this damage is permanent. Nephrotoxic injury causes damage to the epithelium whilst the basement membrane remains intact – this is reversible.

Management of AKI

Clinical management goals for Ronald can be divided into three main categories:

- Restoration of renal perfusion
- Minimising toxic effects
- Correction of metabolic derangements (Davies, 2013)

The immediate issue to be managed is Ronald's severe, potentially life-threatening hyperkalaemia, as his potassium is 6.7 mmol/l. Hyperkalaemia is often a fatal complication in AKI (Davies, 2013). Ronald's failing kidney is unable to excrete potassium effectively as he is not passing urine. Hyperkalaemia presents a very real risk of cardiac arrhythmias and cardiac arrest. High levels of potassium decrease the cardiac action potential and interfere with normal propagation of electrical activity in the heart. Ronald was attached to a cardiac monitor to assess his cardiac rhythm and a 12-lead ECG was recorded. These revealed a sinus rhythm with a slightly elevated rate of 92 bpm but no ECG changes. Ronald was given a slow IV injection of Actrapid insulin and 50% glucose (GAIN, 2014). The insulin acts to push the potassium from the blood back into the cell thereby lowering the serum level of potassium. The glucose is given to offset potential hypoglycaemia. To further monitor this, the nurse also checked Ronald's capillary glucose regularly for the next few hours, and urea and electrolytes (U & Es). Serum potassium levels had reduced to 5.0 mmol/l later in the day.

A review of Ronald's medication identified the nephrotoxic effects of the NSAID he had been taking for many years for his rheumatoid arthritis and this medication was stopped to prevent further potassium accumulation and halt damage to the kidneys.

As the life-threatening problem had been addressed, a more thorough review of Ronald's history and presentation could take place to identify the cause of the AKI and plan his management. His vital signs remained unchanged and he remains on the surgical ward in a bedside that is readily visible to the nursing team.

Ongoing management of AKI

Airway and breathing

Ronald's airway patency presents no present concern as he is able to converse normally. He is maintaining his oxygen saturation within the target 94–98% (BTS, 2017) on room air. His SpO_2 will be monitored a minimum of four hourly to ensure that he maintains this level of oxygen perfusion. The nursing team recognise that with the reduced tissue perfusion he is at risk of developing hypoxia and that the intravenous fluid infusion has a risk of him developing pulmonary oedema if he becomes fluid overloaded. They have also encouraged Ronald to report any difficulties he has with his breathing. He is working quite hard at 20 breaths per minute so they have optimised his position, sitting him upright, well supported by pillows. An arterial blood gas was requested to identify any potential acidosis.

Circulation

In order to restore renal perfusion, Ronald requires intravenous fluids as the cause of his AKI was identified as volume responsive and attributed to hypovolaemia secondary to diarrhoea and vomiting. The surgeons discussed the likelihood of bleeding from the hernia repair site causing the hypovolaemia but concluded there were no clinical indications of this. This fluid challenge would also aid in correcting the electrolyte imbalance and to help him maintain his hydration status. A crystalloid infusion of maintenance fluids using algorithm 3 of the NICE (2013, updated May 2017) intravenous fluid therapy guidelines was commenced. A strict fluid balance chart was implemented to record all input and output hourly, accurately aiming to meet the 0.5ml/kg/hour threshold = 38 mls/hour based on Ronald's pre-admission weight. The patency of Ronald's catheter was confirmed and a catheter specimen of urine was sent for culture and sensitivity as he was now passing small amounts of urine. A ward-based dipstick revealed a small amount of protein but the CSU did not indicate a urinary infection. An anti-emetic was prescribed and administered and as the infusion proceeded the nausea receded and Ronald was encouraged to drink oral fluids. Ronald's nausea and vomiting was due to the accumulation of nitrogenous waste products evident in his elevated urea.

Ronald will also need support with his nutritional intake and was therefore referred to the dietician. Patients with AKI metabolism are under great stress, resulting in the need for extra calories and extra protein (Davies, 2013). A MUST assessment (BAPEN, 2003) was completed to aid in assessment of malnutrition; Ronald may need enteral nutrition to meet his needs in the immediate phase (NICE, 2006, updated 2017). Ronald also had an elevated potassium level and would require dietary advice regarding a diet low in potassium.

Ronald's serum electrolyte results will need to be repeated to see if the fluid challenge sees an improvement in his renal function.

Ronald's four-hourly observations of vital signs and cardiac monitoring will continue to monitor his blood pressure and heart rate, looking for any cardiac arrhythmias or signs of deterioration in his tissue perfusion or fluid overload causing strain on his heart. In addition to monitoring his fluid balance, he will be weighed daily to aid in assessment of oedema and fluid retention. Ronald will need four-hourly temperature monitoring to aid in identification of potential infection.

Disability

ACVPU needs to be undertaken with the NEWS2 scoring. This will demonstrate how effective Ronald's cerebral perfusion is; this is particularly relevant as elevated urea is associated with neurological problems and confusion. Ronald requires regular assessment for abdominal pain, which will likely improve once the vomiting recedes. Paracetamol was prescribed as an analgesic as the NSAID had been discontinued. Blood glucose levels need to be monitored to evaluate the sympathetic nervous system response to this acute illness and follow up the administration of glucose to treat the hyperkalaemia.

Exposure

Ronald requires a 'top-to-toe' examination, maintaining his privacy and dignity. Due to his episode of illness he is at high risk of tissue breakdown and development of a pressure ulcer. A recognised assessment tool such as Braden or Waterlow will help to define his risk and implement pressure relieving measures. Due to his dehydrated state, Ronald's skin was dry and had reduced turgor – this should improve with fluid replacement. Itchy skin and a uraemic rash can also appear due to elevated urea levels and the nurse will also need to be alert to this. Ronald's bowel movements will need to be recorded on a stool chart and a specimen sent for culture and sensitivity, and tested for the presence of blood. In light of the duration of time he has received a NSAID for rheumatoid arthritis, assessment should take place regarding potential irritation to the stomach lining and risk of bleeding.

Monitoring and assessment of Ronald's renal function should continue until it is clear that Ronald has responded to treatment and is safe to be discharged. Preparation for discharge should include a multidisciplinary approach to promote self management including risks related to development of AKI and dietary information and involve family and/or carers as appropriate. It would also be appropriate to provide information about charitable organisations that support people who have experienced AKI.

Conclusion

A case study considering a patient, Ronald Hunt presenting with AKI has been considered, outlining the relevant pathophysiology and incorporating evidence-based interventions and management strategies.

CASE STUDY 7.5: ANAPHYLAXIS – AL WEST

The final and fifth case study in this chapter considers a patient who has an anaphylactic reaction and is at risk of distributive shock. Anaphylaxis is a severe, life-threatening, generalised or systemic hypersensitivity reaction to drugs, toxins, foods or plants characterised by a rapid onset. Pathophysiology underpinning an anaphylactic reaction has been presented in Chapter 6 under discussion of distributive shock.

It is characterised by rapidly developing, life-threatening problems involving: the airway (pharyngeal or laryngeal oedema) and/or breathing (bronchospasm with tachypnoea) and/or circulation (hypotension and/or tachycardia). In most cases, there are associated skin and mucosal changes (NICE, 2011, updated 2020). Box 7.12 identifies signs and symptoms of anaphylaxis presented in a systematic ABCDE assessment. Anaphylaxis can be triggered by any of a very broad range of triggers, but those most commonly identified include food, drugs and venom. Of foods, nuts are the most common cause while muscle relaxants, antibiotics, NSAIDs and aspirin are the most commonly implicated drugs (Resuscitation Council UK (RCUK), 2021). It is important to note that, in many cases, no cause can be identified and that a significant number of cases of anaphylaxis are idiopathic (non-IgE mediated).

Presenting data about the incidence of anaphylaxis in the UK is problematic as despite simplified treatment guidance from the RCUK and NICE on identification and diagnosis, misdiagnosis occurs for example with patients being given treatment for anaphylaxis presenting solely with skin changes, panic attacks or a vaso-vagal episode. There is not a recent evidence base to draw on in this area but it is suggested approximately 1 in 1333 of the population of England has experienced anaphylaxis and that there are approximately 20 deaths a year attributed to anaphylaxis in the UK (NICE, 2011, updated 2020).

Box 7.12 Signs and symptoms of anaphylaxis

Airway

- Swelling of airway (lips, mouth pharynx and larynx), angioedema

(Continued)

Breathing

- Rapid respiratory rate, shallow, using accessory muscles, low SpO_2, metabolic acidosis
- Bronchoconstriction – wheezing, stridor, shortness of breath, coughing
- Excessive mucous production

Circulation

- Very rapid and weak pulse, CRT >2 sec, vasodilation, hypotension

Disability

- Very anxious and restless, elevated glucose level, apprehension, flushing ('impending doom')

Exposure

- Skin and/or mucosal changes – rash, urticaria, flushing, angioedema, cyanosis
- Generalized itching or burning, warm skin

Al's initial observations recorded by the paramedic are in Box 7.13. Compare this history to the signs and symptoms listed in Box 7.12.

Box 7.13 Al's initial observations

Al West is a 35 year old PE teacher. He is usually fit and well. He is taking the school hockey team to a three-day tournament at another school. After the evening meal on the first day of the trip he rapidly starts to feel very unwell. He can feel his lips swelling and tells his colleague that he has difficulty breathing and can feel his heart racing. He has a flushed appearance and a nettle-like red rash has developed over his body. Al's colleague is very worried and calls for an ambulance. Al is carrying an adrenaline injector. Al weighs 65 kgs.

Airway

- Al's lips are swollen
- Paradoxical chest and abdominal movements ('see-saw' respirations) and the use of the accessory muscles of respiration
- Al is able to speak one or two words

Breathing

- Respiratory rate: 30 breaths per minute (bpm), shallow
- Oxygen saturation levels: 92% on air
- Audible wheeze on examination

(Continued)

Circulation

- Blood pressure: 100/60 mmHg
- Heart rate: 140 beats per minute, pulse weak
- Temperature: 36.8°C
- Capillary refill time (CRT): 5 seconds

Disability

- Alert on ACVPU, restless and anxious
- Blood glucose: 7.0 mmol/l

Exposure

- Pressure areas intact
- Generalised urticaria over body, feels warm and appears flushed

Management of anaphylaxis in the UK is driven by two key clinical drivers: the Resuscitation Council UK (2021) *Emergency treatment of anaphylaxis: Guidelines for healthcare providers* and NICE CG134 (2011, updated 2020) *Anaphylaxis: Assessment and referral after emergency treatment*.

Assessment

The Resuscitation Council UK (2021) emphasise the importance of using a systematic ABCDE approach for assessment of patients with suspected anaphylaxis as it immediately addressees the life-threatening problems. If an airway is at risk or occluded this needs to be addressed as the priority – there is no point in moving on to address B, C, D or E if the airway is compromised. Guidelines emphasise that healthcare practitioners must act within their scope of practice using skills that they know and use regularly. This is of importance as many healthcare practitioners may never see anaphylaxis or only see it very infrequently in their career. Keeping up-to-date and competent in assessment in this area is of vital importance.

In this scenario, a swift call for help by Al's colleague has probably saved his life.

In line with defining an anaphylactic response, Al's reaction to an allergen was sudden, developing in a few minutes and was unexpected. Following clinical guidance, Al's management will be considered using an ABCDE structure and assessment and intervention is undertaken by a trained and skilled paramedic.

Airway

On arrival to the scene the paramedic finds Al slumped on the floor, accompanied by his colleague. Whilst waiting for the ambulance, Al has self-administered his adrenaline auto-injector.

Al appears unwell, he is struggling to breathe normally and has a flushed appearance. On asking him 'How are you?', he is able to respond with one or two words. This is very concerning and indicates that Al is critically unwell and that his airway is at risk. The paradoxical chest and abdominal movements referred to as 'see-saw' respirations indicate some airway obstruction as Al attempts to breathe; the diaphragm descends, causing the abdomen to lift and the chest to sink. The reverse happens as the diaphragm relaxes. Al's lips are swollen, indicative of an allergic response causing angioedema. The paramedic assists Al to sit in a more upright position to support his airway and the technician applies monitoring equipment including a pulse oximeter, ECG and non-invasive blood pressure monitor. High flow oxygen at 15l/min using a non-rebreathe mask is applied to avoid hypoxic injury to the vital organs. Continuous reassessment of the airway is vital as tracheal intubation may be needed in anaphylactic shock. See Chapter 3 for detailed discussion of airway assessment and airway adjuncts.

Breathing

Al is tachypnoeic and is only managing to breathe shallowly and there is readily observable use of the accessory muscles of respiration with his shoulders rising up with each breath. Chest expansion was found to be equal although shallow and there was an audible wheeze, indicative of partial airway obstruction both listening at a distance and on auscultation. Wheeze is due to the effects of histamine causing constriction and inflammation of smooth muscles in the airways. The trachea was centrally aligned, indicating a pneumothorax was unlikely. The paramedic was already noting the features consistent with an anaphylactic response from observation of Al and noting the history – the sudden onset and rapid progression of symptoms and the potentially life threatening airway and breathing problems. SpO_2 was recorded at 92% before commencement of high flow oxygen; however the reliability of this peripheral measure in the context of Al's presentation and partial airway obstruction could not be relied upon. In line with Resuscitation Council guidelines (2021), Al was advised to avoid sudden changes in posture and maintain a supine position.

Circulation

Al's body feels warm and a nettle-like urticaric rash is present over the visible parts of Al's body – this is due to histamine release. From observing the cardiac monitor, the paramedic treating Al could see that he was tachycardic although in a sinus rhythm; his pulse was palpable radially but weak and capillary refill time was prolonged. At this point, in line with RCUK (2021), NICE (2011, updated 2020) and RCP (2009) guidance a decision was made to administer a further dose of adrenaline. The earlier this is given the better the clinical outcome (RCP, 2009).

A dose of 500 micrograms of a concentration of 1:1000 was administered intramuscularly. Adrenaline reverses the peripheral vasodilatation by suppressing histamine release, reduces peripheral oedema and reduces bronchospasm. The intramuscular route has been identified as preferred over an intravenous route in non-specialist areas, and as being safer and readily available as a form of access (RCUK, 2021).

Al is at risk of developing a distributive form of shock if the loss of vasomotor tone resulting in altered blood flow is not addressed and his tissue perfusion and blood pressure reduce. Al's body is currently compensating for the reduction in blood flow through the hormonal, chemical and neural mechanisms discussed earlier in the chapter.

After administration of adrenaline and a visible reduction in respiratory rate and effort, the A, B and C were reassessed and Al was moved to the ambulance to complete the initial assessment on route to the local emergency department. Intravenous cannulation was achieved with some difficulty due to the peripheral effects of vasodilation caused by the allergen-mediated response.

On arrival at the emergency department Al was visibly more comfortable but remained highly anxious and distressed about the unfolding event. His vital signs on admission to the emergency department are shown in Box 7.14.

Box 7.14 Al's observations on admission to the emergency department

Airway

- There is some swelling around Al's lips
- Al is able to speak in complete sentences

Breathing

- Respiratory rate: 18 breaths per minute (bpm)
- Oxygen saturation levels: 99% on 15l O_2
- Slight wheeze on examination

Circulation

- Blood pressure: 118/60 mmHg
- Heart rate: 100 beats per minute
- Temperature: 36.8°C
- Capillary refill time (CRT): 2 seconds

(Continued)

Disability

- Alert on ACVPU, anxious
- Blood glucose: 7.0 mmol/l

Exposure

- Pressure areas intact
- Generalised urticaria over body, feels warm and appears flushed

---

Ongoing management

On arrival to the Emergency Department (ED) Al's care was taken over by the ED team. The key priority was to assess and monitor Al, to confirm the diagnosis and monitor for any deterioration. A later calculation of the initial NEWS2 (RCP, 2017) gave a score of 8. In the out of hospital emergency context, calculation of the early warning score was not a priority as the severity of the situation and urgency of response required overrode this. On admission to the ED, Al's NEWS2 score had reduced to 3 indicating Al was still triggering on the early warning criteria and required close monitoring.

Airway and breathing

Patency of Al's airway needs to be carefully monitored for risk of deterioration due to angioedema of the larynx and bronchospasm. Nebulised salbutamol administered whilst he is sitting upright will help with reducing wheeze and bronchospasm. It relieves smooth muscle spasm and increases ciliary transport, allowing more efficient clearance of mucus from the airways. Salbutamol can cause tachycardia so cardiac monitoring of Al needs to continue to observe for any further increase in heart rate.

Al's SpO_2 is now being well maintained on high flow oxygen so this can be titrated down in line with BTS (2017) target oxygen saturations of 94–98%. A venturi type mask would be appropriate so a fixed concentration of oxygen can be administered in line with the BTS (2017) oxygen escalator.

Circulation

In line with RCUK (2021) guidance and NICE (2013, updated May 2017) fluid therapy guidance, an intravenous fluid challenge of 500 mls of crystalloid was administered. The allergic response can cause large volumes of fluid to leak from the circulatory system during a reaction causing a drop in cardiac output and tissue perfusion. Al's blood pressure, reducing heart rate and improving capillary refill indicate that this fluid challenge along with the administration of adrenaline had been effective in reducing the risk of distributive shock. As Al was now more stable, a non-sedating oral antihistamine was administered to alleviate the skin discomfort cause by the urticaria (Resuscitation Council, 2021). Similarly a dose of 200mg hydrocortisone IV was administered slowly – its anti-inflammatory properties may help to shorten the reaction period and reduce the uptake of histamine at H1 and H2 receptor sites (Linton & Watson, 2010).

Cardiac monitoring of Al and regular observation of vital signs need to be continued, a minimum of every 15 minutes in the first hour and ongoing for at least six hours. This is important as in approximately 20% of cases a biphasic (or 'rebound') reaction is observed without further exposure to the allergen (Caton & Flynn, 2013). Pourmand et al. (2018) identify that biphasic reactions have been reported up to 72 hours after initial onset although mortality figures were not influenced by the period of monitoring in the ED. This period of observation will also allow time for effective post-reaction follow up to be implemented.

Disability

ACVPU needs to be undertaken with the NEWS2 scoring. Al is understandably anxious after experiencing this potentially life threatening event and will require effective psychosocial support adhering to the principles of the 6Cs (Cummings & Bennett, 2012).

Exposure

Changes to Al's skin and the presence of an urticaric rash are due to the binding of IgE to the allergen, triggering the release of substances from mast cells that cause inflammation including skin change. This should recede as the reaction subsides but a top-to-toe examination should take place to ensure there has been no skin breakdown. NICE (2011, updated 2020) recommend that after a suspected anaphylactic reaction in adults or young people aged 16 years or older, timed blood samples for mast cell tryptase testing should be taken as follows:

• A sample as soon as possible after emergency treatment has started.
• A second sample ideally within one to two hours (but no later than four hours) from the onset of symptoms.

Al should be offered a referral to a specialist allergy service consisting of healthcare professionals with the skills and competencies necessary to accurately investigate, diagnose, monitor and provide ongoing management of, and patient education about, suspected anaphylaxis (NICE, 2011, updated 2020). Part of this interprofessional approach to treatment would include dietician input as Al had a history of nut allergy and a food trigger may have been the cause of this episode. His adrenaline auto-injector should be replaced, also considering the prescription of more than one injector. Al should be advised to check the expiry date and replace when needed but not to refrain from using it if it is out of date and he experiences symptoms of an anaphylactic reaction.

Before discharge, a healthcare professional with the appropriate skills and competencies should offer (NICE, 2011, updated 2020):

- Information about anaphylaxis, including the signs and symptoms of an anaphylactic reaction.
- Information about the risk of a biphasic reaction.
- Information on what to do if an anaphylactic reaction occurs (use the adrenaline injector and call emergency services).
- A demonstration of the correct use of the adrenaline injector and when to use it.
- Advice about how to avoid the suspected trigger (if known).
- Information about the need for referral to a specialist allergy service and the referral process.
- Information about patient support groups.

In order for the public and healthcare professionals to be aware of Al's risk of anaphylaxis, he should wear some form of alert bracelet/band in addition to making friends and family aware of the signs and symptoms of anaphylaxis.

NICE (2011, updated 2020) guidelines recommend that Al should be observed for 6–12 hours from the onset of symptoms and the RCP (2009) stipulate review by a senior clinician must take place before discharge. Once advice and education has been given and symptoms have sufficiently receded, Al can be discharged home.

The Anaphylaxis Campaign website's 'Healthcare professionals' section contains useful advice that may be used in supporting patients: www.anaphylaxis.org.uk/hcp/

Conclusion

A case study considering a patient, Al West presenting with anaphylaxis has been considered, outlining the relevant pathophysiology and incorporating evidence-based interventions and management strategies.

REFERENCES

Baigent, C., Collins, R., Appleby, P., Parish, S., Sleight, P. & Peto, R. (1998) ISIS-2: 10 year survival among patients with suspected acute myocardial infarction in randomised comparison of intravenous streptokinase, oral aspirin, both, or neither. The ISIS-2 (Second International Study of Infarct Survival) Collaborative Group. *British Medical Journal*, 316 (7141), 1337–1343.

BAPEN (2003) *Introducing 'MUST'*. Available at: www.bapen.org.uk/screening-and-must/must/introducing-must (accessed 20 September 2018).

British National Formulary (BNF) (2022) Diamorphine Hydrochloride. Available at: https://bnf.nice.org.uk/drug/diamorphine-hydrochloride.html (accessed 13 February 2022).

British Heart Foundation (BHF) (2018) *British Heart Foundation UK factsheet*. Available at: www.bhf.org.uk/what-we-do/our-research/heart-statistics (accessed 20 September 2018).

British Thoracic Society (BTS) (2017) *BTS guideline for emergency oxygen use in adults in healthcare and emergency settings*. Available at: www.brit-thoracic.org.uk/standards-of-care/guidelines/bts-guideline-for-emergency-oxygen-use-in-adult-patients/ (accessed 20 September 2018).

Caceres, M., Esmailian, F., Moriguchi, J., Arabia, F. & Czer, L. (2014) Mechanical circulatory support in cardiogenic shock following an acute myocardial infarction: A systematic review. *Journal of Cardiac Surgery*, 29 (5), 743–751.

Caton, E. & Flynn, M. (2013) Management of anaphylaxis in the ED: A clinical audit. *International Emergency Nursing*, 21, 64–70.

Cecconi, M., De Backer, D., Antonelli, M., Beale, R., Bakker, J., Hofer, C., Jaeschke, R., Mebazaa, A., Pinsky, M., Teboul, J., Vincent, J. & Rhodes, A. (2014) Consensus on circulatory shock and hemodynamic monitoring. Task force of the European Society of Intensive Care Medicine. *Intensive Care Medicine*, 40 (12), 1795–1815.

Cummings, J. & Bennett, V. (2012) *Compassion in practice nursing, midwifery and care staff: Our vision and strategy*, Department of Health. Available at: www.england.nhs.uk/wp-content/uploads/2012/12/compassion-in-practice.pdf (accessed 23 September 2018).

Davies, A. (2013) Acute Kidney Injury. In N. Thomas (Ed.), *Renal Nursing* (Ch. 5). Hoboken: John Wiley & Sons.

Francis, R. (2013) *Report of the Mid Staffordshire Public Inquiry, Vols. 1–3*. Available at: www.gov.uk/government/publications/report-of-the-mid-staffordshire-nhs-foundation-trust-public-inquiry (accessed 23 September 2018).

Guidelines and Audit Implementation Network (GAIN) (2014) *Guidelines for the treatment of hyperkalaemia in adults*. Available at: www.rqia.org.uk/RQIA/files/6f/6f51b366-f8bf-44de-a630-6967d5353a87.pdf (accessed 23 September 2018).

Intensive Care Society (ICS) (2009) *Levels of critical care for adult patients*. Available at: www.ics. ac.uk/ICS/guidelines-and-standards.aspx (accessed 23 September 2018).

Léopold, V., Gayat, E., Pirracchio, R., Spinar, J., Parenica, J., Tarvasmäki, T., Lassus, J., Harjola, V. P., Champion, S., Zannad, F., Valente, S., Urban, P., Chua, H. R., Bellomo, R., Popovic, B., Ouweneel, D. M., Henriques, J. P. S., Simonis, G., Lévy, B., Kimmoun, A., Gaudard, P., Basir, M. B., Markota, A., Adler, C., Reuter, H., Mebazaa, A. & Chouihed, T. (2018) Epinephrine and short-term survival in cardiogenic shock: An individual data meta-analysis of 2583 patients. *Intensive Care Medicine*, 44 (6), 847–856.

Lewis, S., Pritchard, M., Evans, D., Butler, A., Alderson, P., Smith, A. & Roberts, I. (2018) Colloids versus crystalloids for fluid resuscitation in critically ill people. *Cochrane Database of Systematic Reviews*, 8 (CD000567). Available at: www.cochranelibrary.com/cdsr/doi/10.1002/14651858. CD000567.pub7/full> (accessed 23 September 2018).

Linton, E. & Watson, D. (2010) Recognition, assessment and management of anaphylaxis. *Nursing Standard*, 24 (46), 35–39.

Mebazaa, A., Combes, A., van Diepen, S., Hollinger, A., Katz, J., Landoni, G., Hajjar, L., Lassus, J., Lebreton, G., Montalescot, G., Park, J., Price, S., Sionis, A., Yannopolos, D., Harjola, V., Levy, B. & Thiele, H. (2018) Management of cardiogenic shock complicating myocardial infarction. *Intensive Care Medicine*, 44, 760–773.

Migliozzi, J. (2017) Shock. In M. Nair & I. Peate (Eds.), *Fundamentals of Applied Pathophysiology: An Essential Guide for Nursing and Healthcare Students*. Chichester: John Wiley & Sons.

National Confidential Enquiry into Patient Outcome and Death (NCEPOD) (1999) *Extremes of age*. Available at: www.ncepod.org.uk/1999report/99full.pdf (accessed 23 September 2018).

National Confidential Enquiry into Patient Outcome and Death (NCEPOD) (2009) *Adding insult to injury*. Available at: www.ncepod.org.uk/2009report1/Downloads/AKI_report.pdf (accessed 23 September 2018).

National Confidential Enquiry into Patient Outcome and Death (NCEPOD) (2015) *Just say sepsis!* Available at: www.ncepod.org.uk/2015report2/downloads/JustSaySepsis_FullReport.pdf (accessed 23 September 2018).

National Confidential Enquiry into Patient Outcome and Death (NCEPOD) (2016) *Treat the cause*. Available at: www.ncepod.org.uk/2016report1/downloads/TreatTheCause_fullReport. pdf (accessed 26 January 2022).

NHS Improvement (2018) *SBAR communication tool – situation, background, assessment, recommendation*. Available at: https://improvement.nhs.uk/documents/2162/sbar-communication-tool. pdf (accessed 23 September 2018).

NICE (2006, updated 2017) *Nutrition support for adults: Oral nutrition support, enteral tube feeding and parenteral nutrition*. Available at: www.nice.org.uk/guidance/cg32 (accessed 27 September 2018).

NICE (2010, updated 2016) *Chest pain of recent onset: Assessment and diagnosis.* Available at: www. nice.org.uk/guidance/cg95 (accessed 10 April 2021).

NICE (2011, updated 2020) *Anaphylaxis: Assessment and referral after emergency treatment.* Available at: www.nice.org.uk/guidance/cg134 (accessed 27 September 2018).

NICE (2013, updated 2017) *Intravenous fluid therapy in adults in hospital.* Available at: www.nice. org.uk/guidance/cg174 (accessed 27 September 2018).

NICE (2015) *Blood transfusion.* Available at: www.nice.org.uk/guidance/ng24 (accessed 27 September 2018).

NICE (2016a, updated 2017) *Sepsis: Recognition, diagnosis and early management.* Available at: www.nice.org.uk/guidance/ng51 (accessed 27 September 2018).

NICE (2016b) *Major trauma: Assessment and initial management.* Available at: www.nice.org.uk/ guidance/ng39 (accessed 27 September 2018).

NICE (2019) *Acute kidney injury: Prevention, detection and management.* Available at: www.nice. org.uk/guidance/ng148 (accessed 10 April 2021).

NICE (2020) *Acute coronary syndromes.* Available at: www.nice.org.uk/guidance/ng185 (accessed 10 April 2021).

NMC (2015, updated 2018) *The code. Professional standards of practice and behaviour for nurses and midwives.* Available at: www.nmc.org.uk/standards/code/ (accessed 10 April 2021).

O'Driscoll, B., Howard, L. & Davison, A. (2008) BTS guideline for emergency oxygen use in adult patients. *Thorax*, 63, Supplement 6, 1–68. Available at: https://thorax.bmj.com/ content/63/Suppl_6/vi1.long (accessed 27 September 2018).

Pourmand, A., Robinson, C., Syed, W. & Mazer-Amirshabi, M. (2018) Biphasic anaphylaxis: A review of the literature and implications for emergency management. *American Journal of Emergency Medicine*, 36, 1480–1485.

Resuscitation Council (UK) (2021) *Emergency Treatment of Anaphylaxis: Guidelines for Healthcare Providers.* London: Resuscitation Council (UK). Available at: https://www.resus.org.uk/library/ additional-guidance/guidance-anaphylaxis/emergency-treatment (accessed 13 February 2021).

Royal College of Physicians (RCP) (2009) *Emergency treatment of anaphylaxis in adults.* Available at: www.rcplondon.ac.uk/guidelines-policy/emergency-treatment-anaphylaxis-adults (accessed 23 September 2018).

Royal College of Physicians (RCP) (2017) *National Early Warning Score (NEWS) 2: Standardising the assessment of acute-illness severity in the NHS.* Available at: www.rcplondon.ac.uk/projects/ outputs/national-early-warning-score-news-2 (accessed 23 September 2018).

Singer, M., Deutschman, C., Seymour, C., Shankar-Hari, M., Annane, D., Bauer, M., Bellomo, R., Bernard, G., Chiche, J., Coopersmith, C., Hotchkiss, R., Levy, M., Marshall, J., Martin, G., Opal, S., Rubenfeld, G., van der Poll, T., Vincent, J. & Angus, D. (2016) The third inter-national consensus definitions for sepsis and septic shock (sepsis-3). *Journal of the American*

Medical Association, 315 (8), 801–810. Available at: https://jamanetwork.com/journals/jama/fullarticle/2492881 (accessed 23 September 2018).

Tait, D. & Hanson, S. (2016) The patient with acute kidney injury. In D. Tait, J. James, C. Willaims & D. Barton (Eds.), *Acute and Critical Care in Adult Nursing* (Ch. 9). London: Sage.

UK Parliamentary and Health Service Ombudsman Enquiry (2013) *Time to act: Severe sepsis rapid diagnosis and treatment saves lives.* Available at: www.ombudsman.org.uk/publications/time-act-severe-sepsis-rapid-diagnosis-and-treatment-saves-lives-0 (accessed 27 September 2018).

UK Sepsis Trust (2017) *The Sepsis Manual 4th Edition 2017–2018.* Available at: https://sepsis-trust.org/wp-content/uploads/2018/06/Sepsis_Manual_2017_web_download.pdf (accessed 27 September 2018).

Ward, D. (2014) Where has the jugular venous pressure gone? *The British Journal of Cardiology*, 21, 49–50.

WHO (2018) *Sepsis.* Available at: www.who.int/sepsis/en/ (accessed 27 September 2018).

Zeitz, C. & Quinn, T. (2010) Reperfusion strategies. In A. Kucia & T. Quinn (Eds.), *Acute Cardiac Care: A Practical Guide for Nurses* (Ch. 21). Oxford: Wiley-Blackwell.

8

DISABILITY – ANATOMY, PHYSIOLOGY AND PATHOPHYSIOLOGY

SARAH MCGLOIN

Chapter learning outcomes

By the end of this chapter you will be able to:

1. Define the term *consciousness*.
2. Outline the organisation of the nervous system.
3. Identify the key components of a nerve cell.
4. Discuss the role of the key structures within the central nervous system.
5. Explain neuro transmission.
6. Explore the collaboration between the nervous system and the endocrine system to maintain homeostasis.
7. Discuss the neuronal–hormonal pathway.
8. Discuss the role of the autonomic nervous system in the acutely ill patient.
9. Outline the pathophysiology of a raised intra-cranial pressure.

Key words

- Consciousness
- Central nervous system
- Peripheral nervous system

(Continued)

- Autonomic nervous system
- Somatic nervous system
- Neurone
- Synapse
- Neurotransmitter
- Intra-cranial pressure (ICP)

INTRODUCTION

Maintaining homeostasis is essential for the cells and the enzymes within the body to function effectively. Homeostasis is when there is a constant internal environment, in relation to the body's biochemistry (pH, carbon dioxide levels and glucose levels) and body temperature. Both the endocrine and nervous systems are responsible for monitoring and responding to changes within and outside the body and maintaining homeostasis. The nervous system is also responsible for behaviours, long and short term memory and working memory, perception, proprioception and voluntary movements. Furthermore, it is also responsible for moving information from one area of the body to another (Tortora & Derrickson, 2017). In the ABCDE assessment, the nervous system is assessed under 'D – disability.'

WHAT IS CONSCIOUSNESS?

Consciousness is the ability of an individual to receive stimuli via their senses and is a state of being aware of physical experiences or mental thoughts. Conscious patients are awake, aware and responsive to their environment (Marcovitch, 2005). The individual will correctly perceive these incoming stimuli and elicit an appropriate response, which can be defined as a motor response. In order to maintain homeostasis using biofeedback and auto-regulatory processes, an adequate level of consciousness is required.

ORGANISATION OF THE NERVOUS SYSTEM

The nervous system is made up of neural tissue. The functional working unit of this system is the neurone. The nervous system is organised into two parts: the Central Nervous System (CNS) and the Peripheral Nervous System (PNS) (Tortora & Derrickson, 2017). These are presented in Figure 8.1.

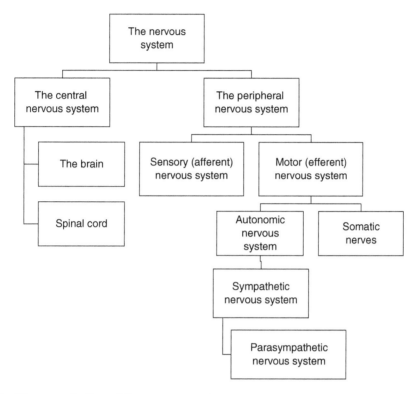

Figure 8.1 The organisation of the nervous system

The neurone

The neurone (presented in Figure 8.2) is the functional unit of the nervous system and is made up of three areas:

1. The dendrite
2. The cell body
3. The axon

The axon and dendrite are also known as *nerve fibres*.

The neurone consists of the cell body, which contains the cytoplasm and nucleus. The cell body is responsible for protein synthesis. They are found tightly packed within the central nervous system and form what is commonly referred to as 'grey matter'. The cell bodies are also responsible for the analysis, integration and storage of information. Because the cell body

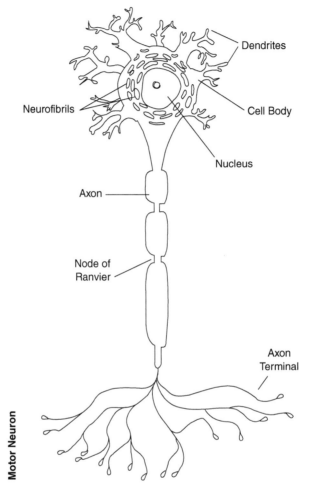

Figure 8.2   A myelinated neurone

does not contain a centrosome, they cannot replicate through mitosis. Because of this, damaged nerve cells through a cerebrovascular accident, acquired brain injury or traumatic brain injury cannot be replaced (Patton & Thibodeau, 2010).

The dendrites are projections from the cell body. They are responsible for receiving information and directing it to the cell body. There can be many dendrites protruding from one cell body (Tortora & Derrickson, 2017). The axon on the other hand is a single projection that transmits information away from the cell body. Axons alter in length and the longer the axon, the longer the neurone and the faster the transmission of information

(Patton & Thibodeau, 2010). At the end of the axon can be a number of axon terminals. These are responsible for connecting with the dendrites of the next neurone in the nerve pathway. One axon can meet with a number of dendrites. This is known as divergence. Alternatively, a number of axon terminals can meet with just one dendrite and this is referred to as *convergence*. Divergence and convergence are important for a nerve pathway to spread out (divergence) or focus back into one point (convergence) (Tortora & Derrickson, 2017). When bundled together, axons form the white matter of the nervous system. The white colour is the result of the myelin sheath that surrounds the nerve fibres.

The functional classification of neurones

Nerve cells can be classified into their function: sensory, integrative or motor neurones (Tortora & Derrickson, 2017). The functional classification of neurones is presented in Table 8.1.

Sensory or afferent nerves

Part of the sensory nervous system, sensory nerves (or 'afferent nerves' as they are sometimes called) transfer information from the peripheral nervous system into the central nervous system. They do this through either the spinal nerves or the cranial nerves. The information they transmit relates to the state of the internal and external environment (Marieb & Keller, 2017).

Interneurons

These are located primarily in the CNS. They form the link between the sensory nerves and the motor nerves (Tortora & Derrickson, 2017).

Motor or efferent nerves

These nerves take information away from the central nervous system to either the muscles or the glands. They bring about an action (or an effect). This could be a muscle moving or a gland secreting a hormone (Marieb & Keller, 2017).

Table 8.1 The functional classification of neurones

Functional classification	Action
Sensory (afferent) nerves	Transmit nerve impulses to the CNS. They monitor internal and external environments and convey this information to the CNS so that it can maintain homeostasis.
Motor (efferent) nerves	Transmit nerve impulses away from the CNS to the muscles, glands and organs of the body. They cause an effect on these structures.
Interneurons	Are located generally within the CNS and form a link between the sensory and motor nerve pathways.

The central nervous system

The central nervous system comprises the brain and the spinal cord. The brain contains a hundred billion neurones. Neuroglial (or glial) cells make up 90% of the cells within the brain (Marieb & Keller, 2017).

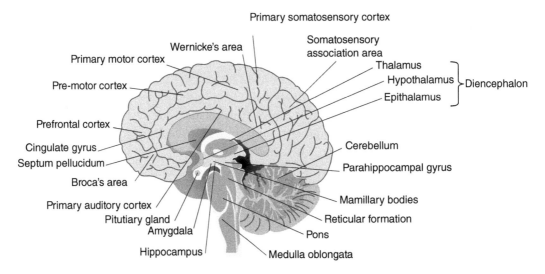

Figure 8.3

The brain composes of six main regions:

1. The medulla oblongata ⎤
2. The pons Brain stem ⎬
3. The midbrain ⎦
4. The diencephalon
5. The cerebrum
6. The cerebellum

The brain stem

This consists of the medulla oblongata, pons and midbrain. It acts as a pathway for nerve impulses travelling between the upper brain and the spinal cord. It also provides the origin for the majority of the cranial nerves (III to XII). The *medulla* contains the cardiac and vaso motor centre, which are responsible for the control of the cardiovascular system. The medulla also contains the reticular activating formation, which is responsible for arousal and awareness; it also controls coughing, vomiting, swallowing, sneezing and hiccoughing. The *pons* controls the rate and depth of breathing through the pneumotaxic and apneustic areas. The *midbrain* is responsible for eye movement, and movement of the head and upper body, in response to painful and auditory stimuli (Tortora & Derrickson, 2017).

The diencephalon

This region of the brain comprises the thalamus and hypothalamus. The *thalamus* acts as a relay station for all the information coming in from the sensory nervous system (apart from smell), and out through the motor nervous system (Tortora & Derrickson, 2017). This region interprets pain, temperature, light, touch and pressure. It is also responsible for emotions and memory.

The *hypothalamus* is responsible for controlling many of the body's vital activities such as hunger, thirst, temperature regulation, sleep (alongside the reticular activating system), emotional behaviour and sexual activity. The hypothalamus also secretes regulating hormones, an example being its regulatory function over the pituitary gland when the hypothalamus regulates the secretion of an anti-diuretic hormone by the posterior pituitary gland when the body needs to conserve water (Marieb & Keller, 2017).

The *limbic system* links together portions of the thalamus, hypothalamus and cerebral hemispheres. These fibre pathways help to control behaviour, emotions, seizures and memory. Other structures in this region include the amygdala (emotions), hippocampus (memory) and pineal gland (sexual activity) (Marieb & Keller, 2017).

The cerebrum

The cerebrum consists of two cerebral hemispheres that are completely separated by the great longitudinal fissure, which includes the corpus callosum (Moini et al., 2021)).

The cerebrum is further split into the four lobes of the brain, which are:

1. The frontal lobe
2. The parietal lobe

3.   The occipital lobe
4.   The temporal lobe

Together these form the higher centres of the brain and are concerned with the interpretation of sensory impulses as well as the control of muscular movement. The cerebrum is also responsible for emotion, intelligence and memory. This includes speech comprehension and production, vision, hearing and skill amongst other things.

The cerebellum

This region controls the subconscious movement of skeletal muscle. This is needed for co-ordination, posture, balance and proprioception (an example being driving whilst adjusting the position of our hands on the steering wheel). The cerebellum is also involved in emotional development and the modulation of both anger and pleasure (Moini et al., 2021).

The meninges

The brain and spinal cord are covered by a series of three layers called meninges. These layers offer protection to the brain parenchyma (Moini et al., 2021) and can be seen in Figure 8.4. There are three meninges:

1.   Dura mater
2.   Arachnoid mater
3.   Pia mater

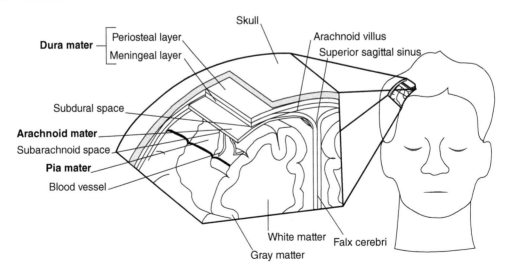

Figure 8.4   The meninges

The dura mater is a continuous double layer of thick fibrous tissue. The outer layer lines the surface of the skull and the inner layer covers the brain and spinal cord. The role of the dura is to stabilise the brain to prevent damage from movement. There is a central area known as the *sagittal sinus,* which contains a large number of blood vessels. This is where blood is collected from the brain parenchyma (tissue) and returned to the heart. There is a potential space between the dura mater and the next layer of meninges. This is known as the *subdural space.*

The arachnoid is a thin layer of connective tissue. The space between this layer and the pia mater is known as the *subarachnoid space* and is filled with cerebral spinal fluid (CSF).

The innermost meninges is the pia mater. This is a thin layer of delicate connective tissue, which covers the surface of the brain and spinal cord. This has a large number of blood vessels. The capillaries of these blood vessels protrude into the brain parenchyma.

The meninges become important when an individual has experienced a brain haemorrhage and are used as markers to describe the location of such bleeds.

Cerebral spinal fluid

The brain is further protected by the cerebral spinal fluid (CSF). This 'straw- like' fluid that is 99% water also contains glucose, proteins, lactic acid, urea and white blood cells, and is produced by the ventricles in the brain.

There are four ventricles within the brain and these are filled with CSF. They are the right and left lateral ventricles, which are the main ventricles and the third and fourth ventricles. The CSF is produced by the Choroid Plexus within the ventricles at a rate of around 500 ml per day. The rate of production matches the rate of reabsorption so the volume of CSF remains constant. The Choroid Plexus forms a network of blood vessels within the ventricles, which deliver nutrients to the brain and remove waste products. They act as a filter by creating a blood–cerebrospinal fluid barrier, which allows certain substances across into the brain and not others. The CSF circulates through the subarachnoid space, around the brain and spinal cord. Its function is to protect the brain by acting as a shock absorber.

The blood supply within the brain

The brain is a highly active part of the body and needs a large amount of oxygen and glucose. The brain receives 15–20% of the cardiac output and uses 20% of the oxygen. The cerebral blood flow will match the brain's metabolic rate, on a supply and demand basis. Consequently, the brain needs a good blood supply. Blood is delivered to the brain by two internal carotid arteries and two vertebral arteries. These all form the circle of Willis. The circle means that the circulation can reach any part of the brain so there is no area left with an inadequate blood supply. The internal jugular veins also return blood from the brain and drain into the subclavian veins.

Intra-cranial pressure and autoregulation of cerebral blood flow

The blood vessels within the brain are able to 'autoregulate' cerebral blood flow. This is achieved by a compensatory mechanism that adjusts the degree of vasodilation and vaso-constriction in response to changes in the cerebral perfusion pressure (CPP). So a decrease in CPP will result in the blood vessels within the brain becoming vasodilated. A raised $PaCO_2$ will also cause the blood vessels to vasodilate whilst a low $PaCO_2$ will cause them to vasoconstrict.

The Munroe–Kellie hypothesis describes the head as being a fixed box (the skull) made up of three components:

1. Blood
2. Brain
3. CSF (Karakis et al., 2017)

The only entrance or exit to this fixed box is at the foramen magnum, which contains the brain stem and respiratory and cardiac centres. To a limited degree these three components are able to compensate themselves for any change in the other components. So for example, if the cerebral blood flow increases, the volume of CSF and fluid in brain tissue can be slightly reduced to compensate. However, if there are large changes in one of the components, this will affect the intra-cranial pressure (ICP). This will then affect the cerebral perfusion pressure (CPP) (Karakis et al., 2017).

CPP is a derived figure and is equal to the mean arterial pressure (MAP) minus the ICP.

CPP = MAP – ICP (mmHg)

When this pressure is too high within the skull, these compensatory mechanisms fail, the CPP falls and the brain may herniate through the tentorium. This is known as 'coning' and has devasting effects on brain stem function, which cause death (Karakis et al., 2017).

The spinal cord

The spinal cord is continuous with the brain stem and exits the cranium at the foramen magnum. The spinal cord is responsible for maintaining homeostasis through the provision of rapid reflex responses to a range of stimuli. The spinal cord carries sensory nerve impulses to the brain. These are known as *ascending nerve pathways* and *motor nerve impulses* – descending nerve pathways away from the brain. There are 31 pairs of spinal nerves that form part of the peripheral nervous system. Each spinal nerve has a dorsal root by which afferent impulses enter the spinal cord and a ventral root by which efferent nerves leave the spinal cord. The dorsal root also acts as a centre for some reflex actions where the brain does not perform interpretation of a sensory impulse. Instead the sensory nerve directly generates a nerve impulse in the motor neurone. An example of this is the spinal knee-jerk reflex (Tortora & Derrickson, 2017).

Cranial nerves

There are 12 pairs of nerves that come from the brain itself. These are referred to as *cranial nerves*. They are responsible for very specialised features and are both named and numbered (Moini et al., 2021). The cranial nerves are presented in Table 8.2.

Table 8.2   Cranial nerves

Cranial nerve		Function
I	Olfractory	Smell
II	Optic	Visual fields and ability to see
III	Occulomotor	Eye movements; eyelid opening; pupil constriction; lens accommodation; proprioception
IV	Trochlear	Eye movements; proprioception
V	Trigeminal	Facial sensation; chewing
VI	Abducens	Eye movements; proprioception
VII	Facial	Eye lid closing; facial expression; saliva; tear secretion
VIII	Vestibularocochlear	Hearing; sense of balance
IX	Glosspharyngeal	Saliva secretion; swallowing; blood pressure regulation
X	Vagus	Visceral muscle movement; swallowing; taste
XI	Accessory	Control of neck and shoulder muscles
XII	Hypoglossal	Speech; swallowing; tongue movement

The peripheral nervous system

The peripheral nervous system consists of all the nervous tissues outside of the CNS. It consists of the somatic nervous system, the autonomic nervous system and the enteric nervous system (ENS). The ENS is the nervous system in the gut. It has been described as the 'brain' of the gut and controls gastrointestinal functions within the body (Tortora & Derrickson, 2017).

The somatic nervous system

Sensory and motor nerves also known as afferent and efferent nerves communicate within the CNS. Motor nerves are voluntary nerves that communicate with skeletal muscle. Sensory nerves on the other hand carry information to the CNS from receptors called 'somatic receptors', which are located throughout the body (Moini et al., 2021).

The autonomic nervous system

The autonomic nervous system (ANS) is involuntary. It controls organs and glands and regulates things such as respiratory rate, heart rate, temperature and blood pressure. It is separated into two parts, the sympathetic nervous system and the parasympathetic nervous system (Tortora & Derrickson, 2017).

Electrical transmission of nerve impulses

Neurones need to communicate with each other and their target tissue in order to have an effect on the body and help to maintain homeostasis. Information from the bodies' external and internal environment is transmitted to the CNS via the sensory nervous system. Once the information reaches the correct area of the brain, the information is then processed and a response is then initiated via the motor nervous system. Such information can be transported either chemically or electrically. The nerve cells are able to generate signals called 'nerve impulses'. These are the electrical signals and are known as *action potentials* (Mayer & Garner, 2009).

An action potential is generated through the movement of ions across the membrane of a neurone. The main ions involved in this are potassium and sodium ions, which are both Cations. Under normal conditions, there are differences in electrical charge across either side of the nerve cell membrane. This is known as a resting potential and the cell is said to be polarised. The resting potential relates to the number of sodium and potassium ions on either side of the nerve cell wall. At rest, the inside of the nerve cell is negative and the outside positive. The inside of the cell has 148 mmol/l of potassium ions and 10 mmol/l of sodium ions, whereas the outside of the cell has 5 mmol/l of potassium ions and 142 mmol/l of sodium. At rest, the cell membrane does not let sodium through – even though it wants to move into the cell via the process of diffusion. But at rest the nerve cell does let potassium slowly diffuse out of the cell by opening up potassium channels in the cell membrane (Mayer & Garner, 2009).

Once a stimulus of adequate strength is applied to the polarised nerve cell, the membrane will depolarise. This is when the cell becomes electrically positively charged on the inside and negatively charged on the outside. Sodium and potassium channels open up in the cell wall and the sodium and potassium rush into the nerve cell. As soon as the inside of the cell becomes positive and the outside negative, the membrane is said to have depolarised and an action potential (or nerve impulse) is generated (Mayer & Garner, 2009).

The action potential is conducted along the axon like a wave. As soon as an action potential has moved from one part of the neurone to another, the previous part of the cell repolarises and stops triggering the nerve impulse. The nerve cell needs to repolarise so that it reaches a state known as the refractory period and is able to then generate another action potential. During the repolarisation period, potassium leaves the cell. However, the cell then needs to get the right concentration of sodium outside the cell and potassium inside the cell for it to return to a resting potential. This is done through a sodium potassium pump where sodium ions are actively transported out of the cell and potassium actively transported into the cell (Mayer & Garner, 2009).

The myelin sheath

Larger axons and the peripheral nervous system neurones are wrapped in a myelin sheath. This insulates the axon and prevents the ions leaking out into the interstitial space, which would reduce the effectiveness of neurotransmission. Between segments of the myelin sheath there are unmyelinated segments known as Nodes of Ranvier (Marieb & Keller, 2017). To increase the speed of transmission, the nerve impulse will move from node to node along an axon. Each time it jumps from a node to the next node, the impulse 'reboots' itself so that the charge remains as fast as it did at the beginning of the nerve fibre. This is known as salutatory conduction. Unmyelinated neurons do not have this and their speed of neurotransmission is not as fast (Marieb & Keller, 2017).

Chemical transmission of nerve impulses

Nerve impulses are transmitted from neurone to neurone across gaps or junctions referred to as synapses. The synapse can be between two neurones or a neuron and an effector cell, which is in an organ, muscle or gland. The activity of the neurone will affect the membrane characteristics of the cell it is synapsing with. For the impulse to move across the synapse, there needs to be chemicals present within the gap. These are known as neurotransmitters (Tortora & Derrickson, 2017).

The synapse between a neurone and another cell type is referred to as a neuro-effector junction (if it is with a muscle cell this may be called a 'neuro-muscular junction'). The pre-synaptic cell and post-synaptic cell are separated by a gap known as the synaptic cleft (Tortora & Derrickson, 2017). This is presented in Figure 8.5.

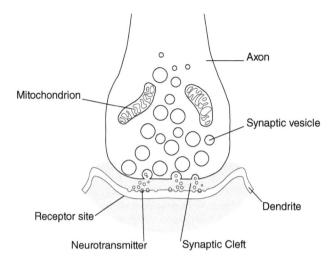

Figure 8.5 The synapse

When a nerve impulse reaches the end of an axon, it comes to an area known as the synaptic cleft. The impulse then triggers the release of a neurotransmitter from the pre-synaptic neurone into the synapse. The neurotransmitter will then diffuse across the gap to the post-synaptic membrane (be this in a skeletal muscle cell, another neurone, endocrine cells or organ cells). The neurotransmitter will then bind with a receptor on the post-synaptic membrane. This will then either excite or inhibit the cell depending on the type of neurotransmitter (Moini et al., 2021). Neurotransmitters then need to be degraded by enzymes or transported back into the pre-synaptic cells. The common neurotransmitters and their actions are presented in Table 8.3.

Table 8.3 The functional characteristics of neurones

Neurotransmitter	Function
Acetyecholine (Ach)	Works at the neuro-muscular junction to activate muscles. This is particularly important for the innervation of the diaphragm during breathing.
Dopamine	Enhances mood, motivation and attention. It also helps regulate movement, attention, learning and emotional responses.
Adrenaline	Flight, fright, fight response by the SNS. Increased heart rate and cardiac output. Pupil dilation. Peripheral vaso constriction but vasodilation to increase blood flow to skeletal muscle tissue.
Noradrenaline	Neurotransmitter of the SNS responsible for vasoconstriction, increasing blood pressure and heart rate.
Gamma Aminobutyric Acid	Inhibitory neurotransmitter reducing neuronal excitability across the nervous system.
Histamine	Responsible for inflammatory response vasodilation and urticaria.
Serotonin	Contributes to feelings of wellbeing and happiness. It regulates cognition, reward, learning, memory and numerous physiological processes.

The endocrine system and the nervous system: The neuronal–hormonal pathway

The endocrine system consists of structures called 'glands', which secrete hormones into the circulation for transport to their target organs. The target organ will have a receptor that the hormone attaches to, stimulating specific physiological changes within the target organ or tissue (Clare, 2011). The endocrine system works closely with the nervous system to manage and co-ordinate other body systems and maintain homeostasis. As seen earlier, the nervous system is responsible for secreting neurotransmitters at the synapse, which has an effect on a specific muscle or gland. The nervous system is responsible for fast and speedy changes whilst the endocrine system acts more slowly through releasing hormones that will have a precise action on the target cells (Tortora & Derrickson, 2017).

Functions of the endocrine system

The endocrine system aims to:

- Maintain homeostasis through regulating metabolism, and fluid and electrolyte balance.
- Control growth and production of cells.
- Control the body's response to external stimuli such as stress.
- Regulate reproduction.
- Integrate and regulate circulatory and digestive activities in collaboration with the ANS. (Clare, 2011)

Hormones

Hormones are found circulating within the blood stream. There are some however called 'paracrines', which act on target cells close by or even within the cell that secreted them without entering the circulation. These are known as autocrines (Clare, 2011).

Hormones are grouped depending upon their structure: polypeptides include hormones secreted from the pituitary gland, pancreas and parathyroid glands; steroids, which are lipid-soluble, are secreted from the adrenal cortex and reproductive glands – these are recognised by ending in 'sterone' (such as progesterone); amines, which are water soluble come from amino acids and include hormones secreted by the thyroid, and catecholamines adrenaline and noradrenaline; and finally eicosanoids, also water soluble, which come from a polyunsaturated fatty acid and include prostaglandins that help mediate the inflammatory response as well as the transmission of pain (Clare, 2011).

The regulation of the nervous system

Hormone secretion is regulated by:

- The hypothalamus, which regulates the release of hormones that have other endocrine glands as their target.
- Rhythmic variations.
- Chemical regulation.
- Neural regulation (Marieb & Keller, 2017).

Hormones are released in response to a specific stimulus, for example low circulating levels of thyroxine stimulate the hypothalamus to secrete thyroid stimulating hormone (TSH), which then in turn stimulates the thyroid to secrete more thyroxine. When the serum levels of thyroxine increase to the desired level, the hypothalamus stops secreting TSH. This is known as a negative feedback system. When the levels of thyroxine drop again, the hypothalamus is 'switched on' again and TSH is once again secreted (Marieb & Keller, 2017).

There are also rhythmic variations over hormone secretion. The adrenocortical hormones follow a 24-hour cycle and link to the circadian rhythm for sleep with secretion of these hormones highest just prior to a person waking up. The menstrual cycle also is an example of this (Clare, 2011).

Chemical regulation happens when endocrine glands are controlled by chemicals and not the pituitary gland. The release of insulin is controlled by a rise in blood glucose levels. When they rise, the pancreas is stimulated to secrete insulin and suppress glucagon. When the blood glucose levels fall, glucagon is secreted and insulin is suppressed (Tortora & Derrickson, 2017).

The focus of this chapter has been disability and the role of the nervous system. The nervous system is also responsible for controlling the secretion of some hormones. This is referred to as the neuronal–hormonal pathway. A key example of this is the release of catecholamines. Adrenaline and noradrenaline are catecholamines and neurotransmitters. They are responsible for controlling blood pressure and heart rate. Their release is under the control of the autonomic nervous system (Marieb & Keller, 2017).

When blood pressure drops, baroreceptors in the aortic arch and carotid sinus stop firing. The cardiac centre in the brain stem senses this and through the sympathetic nervous system (which is part of the autonomic nervous system), the hypothalamus stimulates the adrenal cortex to secrete noradrenaline and adrenaline. These then circulate to the blood vessels where noradrenaline attaches to receptors on the smooth muscle fibres within the blood vessels and causes the blood vessels to constrict. As the blood pressure rises, the baroreceptors start to fire again and the SNS is 'switched off' (Tortora & Derrickson, 2017).

SUMMARY

This chapter has presented the anatomy and physiology of the nervous system. The concept of consciousness has been explored as has the structure of the central nervous system and peripheral nervous system. Neurotransmission has been presented as has the collaboration between the endocrine system and the nervous system. The application of patient-centred approaches to disability will be discussed in the following chapter.

REFERENCES

Clare, C. (2011) The endocrine system. In I. Peate & M. Nair (Eds.), *Fundamentals of Anatomy and Physiology for Student Nurses* (pp. 192–223). Chichester: Wiley-Blackwell.

Karakis, I., Nuccio, A. H., Amadio, J. P. & Fountain, A. J. (2017) The Monro-Kellie doctrine in action: Posterior reversible leukoencephalopathy syndrome caused by intracranial hypotension from lumboperitoneal shunt placement. *World Neurosurgery*, 98 (868), e11–868.e15.

Marcovitch, H. (2005) *Black's Medical Dictionary*. London: Black.

Marieb, E. N & Keller, S. M. (2017) *Essentials of Human Anatomy and Physiology* (12th ed.). Harlow: Pearson.

Mayer, J. & Garner, A. (2009) Action potentials: Understanding generation, propagation and their clinical relevance. *British Journal of Neuroscience Nursing*, 5 (8), 367–371.

Moini, J. Avgeropoulos N.G. and Samsam, M. (2021) *Epidemiology of Brain and Spinal Tunors*. London: Academic Press Elsevier.

Patton, K. T. & Thibodeau, G. A. (2010) *Anatomy and Physiology* (7th ed.). St Lois: Mosby Elsevier.

Tortora, G. J. & Derrickson, B. H. (2017) *Principles of Anatomy and Physiology*. Hoboken: Wiley.

9

PATIENT-CENTRED APPROACHES TO DISABILITY: APPLICATION TO PRACTICE

SARAH MCGLOIN, NATASHA ASCOTT, ALICE SKULL

Chapter learning outcomes

By the end of this chapter you will be able to:

1. Assess a patient using the ABCDE approach.
2. Identify the signs and symptoms of an individual who is experiencing a decreased level of consciousness due to altered neurological status or metabolic changes.
3. Recognise when and how to escalate care.
4. Plan and implement evidence-based care for patients experiencing a decreased level of consciousness.
5. Understand the underlying pathophysiology to those experiencing a decreased level of consciousness.

Key words

- Subarachnoid haemorrhage
- Pain
- Diabetic emergency
- Diabetic keto acidosis (DKA)
- Delirium

INTRODUCTION

This chapter will present four case studies of patients who are experiencing difficulties with their nervous or endocrine system. For each case study, an initial assessment will take place to identify and prioritise the patient's key problems. The underlying pathophysiology will then be explored followed by evidence-based interventions and management strategies for each of the four case studies. The case studies will focus on a decreased level of consciousness following a subarachnoid haemorrhage; a patient experiencing pain; a patient with a diabetic emergency in the form of diabetic keto acidosis (DKA); and a patient experiencing delirium.

Activity 9.1

Read the following case study. Explain what a subarachnoid haemorrhage is.

CASE STUDY 9.1: A DECREASED LEVEL OF CONSCIOUSNESS – SANJEET KAUR

Case study 9.1 takes a look at a patient with a decreased level of consciousness. There may be other causes of a decreased level of consciousness such as alcohol intoxication, recreational drug use or traumatic brain injury. In the case here of Sanjeet Kaur the decreased level of consciousness is the result of a subarachnoid haemorrhage (SAH). This is a type of haemorrhagic stroke when a blood vessel within the brain or on its surface ruptures. SAH accounts for 5% of all strokes and occurs in 2 to 16 people per 100,000 per year (NICE, 2018). In around 80% of people the leak of blood arises from the rupture of an intracerebral arterial aneurysm. Between 10–15% of people with this type of stroke die before reaching hospital (Intercollegiate Stroke Working Party, 2016). Although overall trends show that survival rates are improving, many are left both physically and cognitively impaired. There has been an increase in neurological and neuroscience centres nationally (National Confidential Enquiry into Patient Outcome and Death, 2013). NICE are working on a clinical guideline for the management of patients following a SAH, which was published in 2021.

Case study – Sanjeet's initial assessment

Sanjeet Kaur (42) has been admitted to the Emergency Department complaining of a severe headache towards the back of his head. He is complaining of nausea and his left arm is feeling

(Continued)

weak and difficult to lift up. Sanjeet is a top level lawyer, who works long hours in a stressful environment. He does smoke and when he's not at work he also likes to party hard! He has a girlfriend, but he lives on his own and his parents are his next of kin. On admission, Sanjeet's observations were:

Airway

- Sanjeet was making incomprehensible sounds

Breathing

- Respiratory rate: 8 breaths per minute (bpm)
- Oxygen saturation levels: 85% on air
- Lips and earlobes were cyanosed
- Use of accessory muscles

Circulation

- Blood pressure: 195/87 mmHg
- Heart rate: 121 beats per minute with multiple ectopic beats
- Temperature: 38.2° C
- Urine output: 98 mls/hour over the past hour
- Capillary refill time (CRT): 2 seconds

Disability

- Voice on ACVPU, disorientated to time and place
- Incomprehensible sounds
- Flexing to central pressure
- Pupils left size 8 mm and sluggish; right size 4 mm and reacting to light
- Blood sugar: 7.5 mmol/l

Exposure

- Pressure areas intact

Activity 9.2

Describe the underlying pathophysiology.

Pathophysiology

Cerebral blood flow comes via the aorta. It enters the brain through the internal carotid and vertebral arteries. The circle of Willis sits at the base of the brain. Its circular structure ensures that the cerebral blood supply is able to continue should one of the arteries become occluded.

An aneurysm is a dilation of an artery caused by a weakness in the arterial wall (Marcovitch, 2010). Cerebral aneurysms generally occur at the joins within the circle of Willis or on the large arteries that form the circle of Willis or just branch off from it. Aneurysms form sack-like structures, which resemble a berry on a tree. This is why they are referred to as berry aneurysms.

Most people remain asymptomatic of an aneurysm until the time it ruptures (Hickey & Strayer, 2019). Individuals experience symptoms such as:

- Drooping upper eyelid
- Dilated pupil
- Inability to move eye in a specific direction or the gaze becomes uneven
- Pain above and behind the eye
- Neck pain
- Upper back pain
- Nausea and vomiting (Hickey & Strayer, 2019)

They need to receive urgent care as it could indicate an aneurysm is enlarging and at risk of rupture or has already ruptured. If this is the case, blood rapidly accumulates in the subarachnoid space and may also extend into the brain parenchyma. This will be referred to as an intracerebral haematoma. This will also result in cerebral oedema and a rise in intra-cranial pressure (ICP).

Due to a raised ICP and pressure on the brain stem, Sanjeet's respiratory rate is decreased. This will result in an accumulation of carbon dioxide known as hypercapnia as he is unable to excrete the CO_2 via the respiratory system. This causes a respiratory acidosis. Carbon dioxide is also a powerful vasodilator, which in Sanjeet's case has resulted in the cerebral blood vessels dilating, the cerebral blood flow increasing which in turn has caused his ICP to rise and his cerebral perfusion pressure (CPP) to drop.

Sanjeet is severely hypertensive. This is a compensatory mechanism by the body to try to increase the CPP. CPP is the driving *force pushing blood into the brain* and helps provide oxygen and nutrients to brain tissue. It is calculated by:

CPP = Mean Arterial Pressure (MAP) – ICP
(Hickey & Strayer, 2019)

Management

Sanjeet has had a haemorrhagic stroke in the form of a subarachnoid haemorrhage (SAH). Based upon the Royal College of Physicians' (RCP) *National guidelines for stroke* (RCP, 2016), an immediate computerised tomography (CT) brain scan needs to be organised or better still a CT angiography if possible (RCP, 2016). Sanjeet requires immediate referral to the regional neurosciences centre. However, in the meantime an ABCDE approach to assessment and management needs to be adopted (Resuscitation Council UK, 2015) in the district general hospital where he currently is.

Airway

Sanjeet's airway is patent but at severe risk. The airway needs to be closely monitored and, if there is any further deterioration, care needs to be escalated immediately to the anaesthetic team for advanced airway support. It may be helpful to place an oropharyngeal airway in at this point if Sanjeet will tolerate this, to help protect the airway. Sanjeet needs to be placed in the supine position with his head positioned at 30° which helps reduce ICP and aspiration. His chin should line up with his sternum to help blood flow from the brain.

Breathing

Sanjeet is hypoventilating. This will result in a respiratory acidosis due to his decreased level of consciousness, and poor quality of ventilation. His level of consciousness is reduced and he is unable to compensate for the respiratory acidosis. Sanjeet's oxygen saturations are also very low and he has hypoxaemia. High flow oxygen is administered through a non-rebreathe mask initially. This will be transferred to a humidified fixed oxygen therapy system such as a venturi mask, once ABG readings are taken and analysed. Sanjeet will be at risk of developing a pneumonia due to his decreased level of consciousness and his inability to cough and clear his chest. Therefore oxygen needs to be heated and humidified at all times to prevent atelectasis, basal collapse and pneumonia. Sanjeet should be referred to the physiotherapist for chest physio. At this point he will need referral to the critical care outreach team and anaesthetist for advanced respiratory support.

Circulation

Sanjeet has extreme hypertension, which could be exacerbating his bleed. Rebleeding is associated with an increased risk of mortality and morbidity (Connolly et al., 2012). Sanjeet therefore needs to have an arterial line in situ to enable continuous blood pressure monitoring. Hypertension should be managed with a titratable intravenous anti-hypertensive drug. The Royal College of Physicians' (RCP) *National guidelines for stroke* (RCP, 2016) suggest a target systolic blood pressure of less than 160 mmHg. These drugs may be administered through a central venous access line (CVP line). In line with the guidelines Sanjeet will require 60mg nimodipine four hourly to reduce vasospasm (RCP, 2016). This may need to be administered intravenously and intravenous fluids may need to be commenced. However, it is important to maintain a good CPP. Without ICP monitoring, it is advised to keep the MAP above 90 mmHg, which assumes the ICP is 20 mmHg, and results in a CPP of 70 mmHg (Hickey & Strayer, 2019).

Disability

The RCP guidelines (2016) recommend 'frequent' neurological observations to monitor for signs of deterioration. They do not state how frequent. It is advisable to follow the NICE guidelines for head injury assessment and early management (2019) and record neurological observations:

- Half-hourly for two hours
- Then one-hourly for four hours
- Then two-hourly thereafter

However, should the patient with GCS equal to 15 deteriorate at any time after the initial two-hour period, observations should revert to half-hourly and follow the original frequency schedule.

Should Sanjeet develop any of the following, he will require urgent escalation to the medical team or the critical care outreach team:

- Agitation or abnormal behaviour.
- A sustained (that is, for at least 30 minutes) drop of one point in GCS score (particularly a one-point drop in the motor response score of the GCS).
- Any drop of three or more points in the eye-opening or verbal response scores of the GCS, or two or more points in the motor response score.
- Development of severe or increasing headache or persisting vomiting.
- New or evolving neurological symptoms or signs such as pupil inequality or asymmetry of limb or facial movement.

Neurological observations

Neurological observations (often shortened to 'neuro obs') are a collection of findings relating to the function and integrity of a patient's central nervous system. There are a variety of tools used to support neurological observations within clinical practice including ACVPU and the Glasgow Coma Scale (GCS). Neurological observations are undertaken in three areas:

1. ACVPU or GCS
2. Focal signs: Pupillary response and limb power
3. Vital signs (Derbyshire & Hill, 2018)

ACVPU

Sanjeet's conscious level should be initially assessed using the ACVPU scale (presented in Box 9.1). ACPVU was introduced in NEWS2 (Royal College of Physicians, 2017) and is an updated version of the AVPU scale. Being easier to recall, it is a simplification of the GCS. The main change in this approach is the inclusion of assessment for new-onset confusion. In instances where it is unclear if confusion is new or long standing, it needs to be considered new until proven otherwise. This is a sign of potentially serious clinical deterioration in patients and especially those with confirmed or suspected sepsis (RCP, 2017). New confusion scores 3 on the NEWS2 and the patient will require escalation for urgent assessment.

Box 9.1 The ACPVU scale (RCP, 2017)

- **Alert**: a fully awake patient. Such patients will demonstrate spontaneous eye opening, respond to voice and have motor function. Scores 0 on the NEWS2.
- **Confusion**: a patient may be alert but also confused or disorientated. It is not always possible to determine whether the confusion is 'new' when a patient is acutely ill. Such a presentation should always be considered to be 'new' until confirmed to be otherwise. New-onset or worsening confusion, delirium or any other altered mentation should always prompt concern about potentially serious underlying causes and warrants urgent clinical evaluation. Acute alteration in mentation or new confusion now scores 3 NEWS points as this can be indicative of serious risk of clinical deterioration, especially sepsis.
- **Voice**: the patient makes some response when you talk to them, which could be eyes opening, a verbal response or a motor response – e.g. patient's eyes open on being asked 'Are you okay?'. The response could be as little as a grunt, moan, or slight movement of a limb when prompted by voice. Scores 3 on the NEWS2.
- **Pain**: the patient makes a response to a pain stimulus. A patient who is not alert and who has not responded to voice is likely to only withdraw, have involuntary flexion or extension of the limbs from a painful stimulus. Scores 3 on the NEWS2.
- **Unresponsive**: is also referred to as 'unconscious'. This is if the patient does not give any eye, voice or motor response to voice or pain. Scores 3 on the NEWS2.

Sanjeet is eye-opening to voice but making incomprehensible sounds. In line with NEWS2 he is scoring 3 for neuro and assessment needs to progress to a full GCS and focal signs being recorded.

CASE STUDY 9.2: PATIENT IN ACUTE PAIN AND PAIN ASSESSMENT – STANLEY SMITH

Pain can be classified in various ways but for the purpose of this chapter the term acute pain will be used to incorporate both nociception and neuropathic pain.

Nociception is a normal physiological response to an acute injury or stimulus associated with tissue damage. When it arises from visceral organs such as the bowel or pancreas then it can be referred to as visceral pain whereas pain arising from bone, muscle and connective tissue can be referred to as somatic pain.

Neuropathic pain is a response to abnormal sensory input and can be peripherally generated as in diabetic neuropathy or nerve injury following surgery or centrally generated as in phantom limb pain or spinal cord injury. Neuropathic pain can be a component of acute pain as well as persistent pain and should therefore be part of the assessment process.

For the acutely unwell patient, pain can be an intrinsic part of the body's warning system allowing for early detection and diagnosis. Conversely, poorly managed pain becomes an unpleasant experience for the individual and can have a detrimental effect on various systems throughout the body.

Nociception will trigger both an inflammatory and stress response in addition to an increase in sympathetic activity. This can compromise an individual's recovery and have a profound impact on their psychological wellbeing, increasing the risk of acute pain becoming persistent pain. See Table 9.1 for more information regarding the impact of unrelieved acute pain.

Table 9.1 The impact of unrelieved acute pain

System	Physiological response	Impact on the patient
Cardiovascular system	Increase sympathetic nerve activity	Risk of cardiac ischemia especially if there is pre-existing disease
	Increase in heart rate	
	Increase in contractility	
	Increase in blood pressure	
	Increase in myocardial oxygen demand	
	Decrease in myocardial oxygen supply	

(Continued)

Table 9.1 (Continued)

System	Physiological response	Impact on the patient
Respiratory system	Inability to take deep breaths Reluctance to cough Decrease in residue capacity	Risk of atelectasis and ventilation-perfusion abnormalities Risk of hypoxaemia Risk of pulmonary complications
Gastrointestinal	Decrease in gastrointestinal motility	Risk of ileus, nausea and constipation
Metabolic Immunological Endocrine (Stress response)	Suppression of cellular and immune function Increase in muscle breakdown/catabolic state Hypercoagulation state	Increase risk of infection Prolonged healing Prolonged rehabilitation Increase risk of thromboembolism (DVT and PE)
Psychological wellbeing	Sustained nociceptor input may alter pain perception	Increase in anxiety Poor sleep hygiene Changes in mood and emotion Loss of control and patient autonomy Increased risk of persistent pain

For effective pain management there needs to be an understanding of the pain mechanisms, a comprehensive pain assessment and an appropriate treatment plan titrated to the individual. Regular reassessment is paramount as part of the management to evaluate the treatment outcomes, titrate analgesia and observe for any changes in the clinical picture. The following case study will demonstrate how these principles can be applied in practice.

Box 9.2 Stanley's initial assessment

Stanley is a 67 year old gentleman who was admitted 24 hours ago to the medical assessment unit following a road traffic accident. He has sustained multiple rib fractures 3–6 on his right side. He is known to have hypertension, which is controlled with medication and he was smoking 20 cigarettes a day up until 2 months ago.

Airway

- Stanley appears distressed and mildly confused

(Continued)

Breathing

- Respiratory rate: 22 breaths per minute (bpm), regular but very shallow in nature
- Oxygen saturation levels: 90% on air
- Short of breath and unable to complete his sentences
- Unable to take a deep breath or cough

Circulation

- Blood pressure: 117/56 mmHg
- Heart rate: 90 beats per minute
- Temperature: 38° C

Disability

- Alert on ACVPU, orientated to time and place
- Blood sugar: 6.5 mmol/l
- Right sided chest pain 5/10

Exposure

- Pressure areas intact
- Very reluctant to mobilise

Morbidity and mortality from fractured ribs is often underestimated with a significant increased risk with patients over the age of 65 years and the presence of three or more rib fractures. For every increase in the number of ribs fractured, mortality increases by 19% while the risk of pneumonia increases by 27% (Bulger et al., 2000). For Stanley, both his age and being an ex-smoker will put him in the 'at risk' category.

Pain assessment

The perception of pain is multidimensional, influenced by a combination of physiological, psychological and social factors, making them unique to the individual. Pain assessment is subjective, making self-reporting still the most reliable method of pain assessment. When a patient is unable to communicate, such as when sedated, unconscious or cognitively impaired, self-reporting is no longer reliable or conducive. In these circumstances, pain tools can be used that focus on the behavioural response to pain, such as the Abbey Pain Tool or PAIN AD both commonly used for individuals with dementia, or in more acute environments, the critical care pain observation tool (CPOT) can be used for sedated and/or ventilated patients (Gelinas et al., 2006). It is important to note that when using behavioural tools to assess pain the inclusion of the patient's vital signs is not taken in isolation but taken into account as part of the overall pain assessment. For acute pain there is a common expectation that there will always be an elevated heart rate and blood pressure reading or a change in posture or facial expression. However, physiological, pharmacological and behavioural adaptation can occur, masking signs of pain (Pasero & McCaffery, 2011).

For patients who are able to self report there are several validated pain tools available but the numerical rating score (NRS) is usually the tool of choice for acute pain, e.g. numerical scale ranging from 0 to 3 out of 3, or 0 to 10 out of 10, with 0 being equivalent to no pain and the higher number equivalent to the most severe pain score. The choice of pain tool used will depend on the preferences within the clinical area. What is important to remember is that the choice of tool should remain consistent between clinical areas especially when transferring patients.

The advantage of the NRS is its perceived simplicity and application; however it also has its limitations. Like the behavioural tool it also needs to be used in context, as the concept of using just a number to represent an individual's pain provides no useful information about the nature and characteristics or the underlying mechanism of pain. Although the use of pain tools have been validated in practice they pose their own challenges to pain assessment by the healthcare professionals in their implementation, application and interpretation of the outcome. This can be due to common misconceptions held by healthcare professionals.

For example, if the response to pain by a patient is disproportionate to the expectations held by the healthcare professionals or there is a misconception regarding addictive behaviour then judgements can be made that create barriers to good pain assessment, leading to the poor management of pain.

Without a robust assessment and adequate information, it becomes very difficult to make decisions regarding a patient-centred treatment plan.

Using a framework such as SOCRATES – which is an acronym for Site of pain, Onset, Character, Radiates, Associated symptoms, Time duration, Exacerbating or alleviating factors and Severity – provides a structure to score the severity of pain.

It helps to provide further information regarding an individual's experience of pain as well as an opportunity to build on the relationship between patient and healthcare professional. Managing patients' expectations and providing reassurance at this point is intrinsic to the overall pain management and will help to relay some of the fears and anxieties held by the individuals. Patients' Ideas, Concerns and Expectations (ICE) is an acronym used in general practice (Matthys et al., 2009) but could be incorporated here or used as a prompt to aid the overall assessment.

For Stanley, self-reporting is still the most appropriate form of pain assessment even with his mild confusion. However, an initial assessment should be made to establish the patient's acuity and determine if any immediate action is required for protecting patient safety before a more detailed pain assessment is performed. Here it would be appropriate to administer oxygen therapy for the symptoms of hypoxia before continuing. It would also be appropriate to administer an analgesic to manage the immediate situation. Stanley would be more comfortable and able to breathe and speak before taking a full pain history and planning a more long-term strategy for managing his pain.

Table 9.2 shows an example of an assessment of Stanley's pain using the SOCRATES framework. For measuring the severity of pain a NRS of 0–10 has been used and has been recorded for both static and dynamic pain. This provides a realistic measurement, as Stanley needs to be able to take a deep breath, cough and mobilise to recover and reduce the risks of further deterioration.

Table 9.2 The application of SOCRATES for Stanley

Site	Stanley reports pain in his chest area mainly on the right side, back and shoulders.
Onset	Pain in the chest came on immediately following the incident but the pain in the shoulders and back has been progressive in the last 24 hrs.
Character	Constant dull ache with intermittent severe sharp pain.
	No characteristics at this point to suggest neuropathic pain, i.e. burning, shooting or reports of any altered sensation.
Radiates	Pain radiates into his right shoulder. This is common if there has been an impact on the diaphragm.
Associated symptoms	Difficulty in breathing as it is too painful. Feels fatigued and anxious that he cannot communicate due to his shortness of breath. Has not slept since admission.
Time duration	Continuous dull ache with a rapid onset of severe sharp pain on movement and coughing. The pain does not quickly resolve after the event.
Exacerbating/alleviating factors	Breathing, coughing and movement make the pain worse. The administration of morphine, which has been given, has helped but is not lasting between prescribed doses. This suggests the pain is responding to an opioid but he needs it on a more regular basis.
Severity	A NRS has been used between 0–10.
	At rest, Stanley scores 5/10.
	On movement, 10/10. Ensuring scores are measured for both static and dynamic pain gives a clearer picture of why Stanley is reluctant to take a deep breath, cough and mobilise.

Management

Multimodal analgesia is deemed best practice for managing acute pain. This means a combination of analgesics and analgesic techniques. The aim is to provide the optimum in pain management with the lowest incidence of side effects and adverse reactions. For severe pain, strong opioids are the appropriate drug of choice with consideration to the route of administration. This will vary depending on the outcome of the pain assessment, the individual patient, contraindications and the clinical environment.

Stanley requires a strong opioid for his pain and because the pain increases in severity on movement and taking a deep breath the mode of administration needs to be delivered frequently and have a fast onset. The intravenous route is the most efficient for severe acute pain as it allows for rapid titration and is ideal for a short duration. Stanley is cared for in a clinical area where the staff are trained to manage patients with Patient Controlled Analgesia (PCA). Therefore after being educated in how to use the PCA it will provide safe, effective pain relief for patients with rib fractures and also have the advantage of allowing the patient an element of control. However strong opioids can have unpleasant side effects including sedation, respiratory depression and nausea. Therefore the dose needs to be titrated to the individual and additional opioid sparing analgesics need to be administered regularly. Opioid sparing analgesics are drugs that when administered alongside an opioid will provide an analgesic effect by an alternative mechanism and therefore reduce the need for a higher dose of opioid. Both non-steroidal anti-inflammatory drugs (NSAIDS) and paracetamol are considered to be opioid sparing. If not contraindicated, these should be administered alongside the strong opioid for a syngesic effect. Medication to manage the side effects should be prescribed, including an opioid antagonist such as naloxone to reverse sedation and respiratory depression. Anti-emetics are also important here. If a patient is to be on an opioid for a length of time, laxatives should be considered.

If the pain assessment indicates an element of neuropathic pain then the pain is less likely to respond to opioids and will require neuropathic analgesia, such as gabapentin or pregabalin (Dauri et al., 2009). Tricyclic antidepressants such as amitriptyline may not be appropriate for acute pain because of their slow onset.

There are situations when the side effects of the analgesics outweigh the analgesic benefits as could be possible in Stanley's case. Here adjuvant analgesia and techniques are implemented and will involve other members of the interprofessional team including the anaesthetic and pain team. Consideration will need to be given as to whether the patient needs to be moved to a different environment where they can be monitored more closely by appropriately trained staff. Adjuvant analgesia for acute pain can include local anaesthetic nerve blocks or intravenous lidocaine infusions as well as drugs such as ketamine. Ketamine is an n-Methyl-D-Aspartate (NMDA) receptor antagonist and has been found to have an opioid sparing effect and be effective in managing neuropathic pain (see Table 9.3 for examples of pharmacological interventions for acute pain). For Stanley, a thoracic paravertebral block or a thoracic epidural could be used as an adjuvant as it has proved beneficial in the management of fractured ribs. The localised block would allow him to take a deep breath and cough and therefore able to complete his chest exercises in turn reducing the risks of further complications. Because pain is complex and multidimensional, the different mechanisms of the drugs and techniques used make for efficient multimodal management of acute pain.

Table 9.3 Examples of pharmacological interventions used for acute pain

Group	Medication	Important side effects to consider in the acute phase
Strong opioids	Morphine sulphate	Sedation
	Fentanyl	Respiratory depression
	Oxycodone	Nausea
		Piritus
		Urinary retention
		Constipation
		For prolonged use there would be additional concerns and therefore recommend further reading
Opioid sparing analgesics	Paracetamol	The most serious concern is hepatic toxicity, but this is of minimal risk in individuals with no contraindications and with correct dosing
	NSAIDs (Nonselective COX)	Gastric effects: can vary from gastric irritation to the risk of bleeding and perforation within the gastric tract with prolonged use
	Ibuprofen Naproxen	Renal effects: patients should be assessed for risk factors and comorbidities before use
	Ketorolac Diclofenac	Hematologic effects: as in a possible increase in bleeding time
	(Cox 2 selective)	Cardiovascular effects: patients should be assessed for risk factors and comorbidities before use
	Etoricoxib Celecoxib	Hypersensitivity to respiratory reactions mainly asthmatics
	Parecoxib	N.B. There are serious adverse effects associated with the use of NSAIDs but they still remain beneficial in the management of acute pain, therefore an assessment should always be made on an individual basis. In this scenario an NSAID is not for prolonged use and therefore requires regular review.
Neuropathic agents	Gabapentin	Sedation
Can also be opioid sparing and labelled as adjuvants	Pregabalin	Dizziness
		Somnolence

(Continued)

Table 9.3   (Continued)

Group	Medication	Important side effects to consider in the acute phase
Adjuvant analgesics and techniques Requires an interprofessional team approach. Consideration needs to be given for the patient to be monitored in an environment where staff are trained to manage such techniques	Ketamine	Hypotension or hypertension Hallucinations Sedation Nausea and vomiting Tonic/clonic movements
	Intravenous lidocaine	Nausea and vomiting Abdominal pain Perioral numbness
	Nerve blocks including: thoracic epidurals and thoracic paravertebral blocks	Side effects will be specific to the type of block used. It will depend on where the block is and what drugs have been used in the infusion N.B. Local anaesthetics can be toxic and therefore it requires specialist knowledge to prescribe and implement techniques using this group of drugs

Reassessment

Even once a pain management strategy has been implemented, it is important that regular reassessment takes place. This allows for optimisation and titration. Patients are uniquely individual and the clinical picture can change so it may take time to get it right. Overall what is of paramount importance is the recognised need to manage acute pain to prevent individual suffering and stop further complications of unrelieved pain. Robust pain assessment, early appropriate intervention and involving other members of the interprofessional team are all key and remain the responsibility of everyone looking after the patient.

Activity 9.3

Read the following case study. What is the difference between diabetic ketoacidosis (DKA) and hyperosmolar hyperglycaemic state (HSS)?

CASE STUDY 9.3: DIABETIC KETOACIDOSIS – ROSIE WINTERS

Case study 9.3 takes a look at Rosie Winters (20), a patient experiencing a diabetic emergency. There are a range of conditions that constitute a diabetic emergency including hyperosmolar hyperglycaemic state (HHS) and diabetic keto acidosis (DKA). DKA is associated with Type I diabetes and HHS with Type II but they are both the result of insulin deficiency. In the case here, Rosie is experiencing DKA.

Box 9.3 Rosie's initial assessment

Rosie Winters (20) has been admitted to your ward having experienced vomiting and retching for the past two hours. Rosie has Type I diabetes, which is well controlled; however she does need additional insulin during her monthly menstrual cycle and she is currently on day one of menstruation.

Airway

- Rosie was able to speak in sentences. Her airway was therefore clear

Breathing

- Respiratory rate: 29 breaths per minute (bpm), which are deep and laboured
- Oxygen saturation levels: 100% on air
- Chest clear on auscultation
- Arterial blood gas results showed:
    - pH. 7.31
    - PaO_2 10 kPa
    - $PaCO_2$ 3.3 kPa
    - HCO_3 –7 mmol/l
    - BE –8
    - Lactate 5 mmol/l
    - SaO_2 100%

Circulation

- Blood pressure: 110/65 mmHg
- Heart rate: 120 beats per minute
- Temperature: 37.4° C

(Continued)

- Urine output: 200 mls in the past hour
- Capillary refill time (CRT): 3 seconds

Disability

- Alert on ACVPU but agitated
- Pain score 2/3 with complaints of abdominal pain and headache
- Blood sugar: 26 mmol/l

Exposure

- Pressure areas intact
- Lips were dry and cracked
- Dry skin with increased turgor
- Sunken eyes
- Dry tongue and lips

Activity 9.4

Describe the underlying pathophysiology.

Pathophysiology

To understand the pathophysiology of DKA, you first need to understand normal glucose metabolism and maintenance of blood sugar levels. Glucose is a principal fuel source, which comes mainly from ingested food. The glucose is absorbed through the small intestine and circulates to the hepatic portal vein. Hepatocytes, which are cells in the liver, absorb a lot of the glucose and convert it into its stored form of glycogen. Glycogen is stored in the liver and is reconverted into glucose when blood glucose levels drop.

When glucose is first absorbed there is a spike in blood glucose levels. The beta cells of the pancreas detect this and insulin is secreted. The control of blood glucose levels are regulated by the Islets of Langerhans cells in the pancreas. Insulin stimulates the cells especially in fat and muscle to take up glucose from the circulation and store it until it is required at a later time.

Several hours after eating, blood glucose levels drop as does the insulin level. Glucagon is then released by the alpha cells of the pancreas. Glucagon breaks down the stored form of glucose in the liver called 'glycogen'. Glucagon therefore increases blood sugar levels whilst insulin reduces them (Gosmanov et al., 2014).

Diabetes is a metabolic disorder related to glucose metabolism (Roberts et al., 2015). There is Type I and Type II diabetes. Type I diabetes is an autoimmune disease that destroys the beta cells of the Islets of Langerhans, which prevents insulin from being produced by the pancreas. This results in blood sugar levels increasing. Type II diabetes however sees the pancreas secrete some insulin but this is not enough. Type II diabetes also involves the cells becoming resistant to the insulin or both. Genetics, environmental factors, age, diet and obesity are thought to influence Type II diabetes (Bostock-Cox, 2017). In severe cases patients can experience a diabetic emergency. DKA and HSS are hyperglycaemic emergencies and relate to insufficient insulin production and also an increase in the counter-regulatory hormones including glucagon and cortisol as well as insulin resistance at the cells.

The cells are not getting enough glucose and then start to fail, they can't produce energy in the form of ATP. The cells' inability to function is detected by the body, which thinks there is a lack of circulating glucose, stimulates the liver, adipose tissue and muscle to release their stored forms of glucose. This then increases the blood sugar levels up even further, which with the absence of insulin, still does not enter the cells. This can be known as 'starvation in the face of plenty'. Hyperglycaemia results.

The signs and symptoms of DKA include:

- Hyperglycaemia
- Hyperosmolality
- Ketoacidosis
- Hypovolaemia
- Electrolyte imbalance
- Severe intracellular dehydration

The acidosis seen in DKA is the result of free fatty acids. As adipose tissue breaks down to release more glucose, fatty acids are also released. These are then converted into acidic ketone bodies, which causes the body's pH to drop and to become acidotic and hyperglycaemic.

Hyperglycaemia also causes the blood osmotic pressure to rise. This results in fluid being drawn from the cells and tissues into the blood and circulated to the kidneys. At the same time, due to the hyperglycaemia, the glucose threshold is reached at the nephron and some glucose tips over into the urine. This causes glucosuria and the urine becomes hyperosmotic. This then draws even more water from the circulation into the urine where it is excreted. This results in an excessive production of urine known as polyuria, which can also lead to hypovolaemia. The fluid balance becomes grossly negative as more fluid is being excreted that is being drunk by the patient – especially as in a case like Rosie's where she is already vomiting. Additionally, because the fluid is sitting in the blood and not in the cells, the cells then become dehydrated.

Rosie was diagnosed with DKA because she had a rapid deterioration and a history of Type I diabetes with:

- A blood glucose level >8 mmol/l (Hyperglycaemia)
- A pH less than 7.30 (Acidosis)
- A bicarbonate level 18 mEq/l (Metabolic acidosis) (Farsani et al., 2017)

In contrast, HHS is also characterised by hyperglycaemia and severe dehydration in patients but this time with Type II diabetes. In HHS there is minimal breakdown of adipose tissue and thus ketone bodies being released to cause a ketoacidosis. HHS used to be known as hyperosmolar, non-ketotic syndrome (HONK) but was renamed due to a few patients with Type II diabetes experiencing a degree of ketoacidosis (Lindner et al., 2018). In HHS, because there is not generally an acidosis, the patient collapses due to hypovolaemia (Lindner et al., 2018).

Management

Rosie has been diagnosed with DKA, has lost fluid through vomiting and has not been eating or drinking. Her DKA has been exacerbated by her being on day one of her menstrual cycle, which is also known to increase her blood glucose levels. Rosie's management on the ward followed the NICE National Guideline 17 (2016) *Type I diabetes in adults: Diagnosis and management*. NICE (2016) comments that healthcare professionals managing someone with DKA should be adequately trained with regular updating and be familiar with all aspects of management as presented in Box 9.4.

Box 9.4 Aspects of DKA management in acute care (NICE, 2016)

Fluid balance

Acidosis

Cerebral oedema

Electrolyte imbalance

White cell count; temperature; ECG

Respiratory distress syndrome

Cardiac abnormalities

Precipitating causes

Infection management

Gastroparesis

High dependency and critical care

Airway

Ensure the airway remains patent at all times. Rosie's airway is currently patent as she is able to verbalise; however it will require frequent assessment especially if she deteriorates. Should this occur, Rosie may need additional interventions to maintain her airway patency such as positioning and suctioning. If Rosie's condition deteriorates further and she is unable to maintain her airway, an airway adjunct may be necessary.

Breathing

Ensure Rosie's oxygen saturation levels remains greater than 94% (RCP, 2018). High flow oxygen may be required if her saturation levels fall below this level. Monitor arterial blood gas results regularly during the acute phase, paying particular attention to the pH, lactate and base excess as this will indicate if fluid therapy has been effective and peripheral circulation has been restored, and the metabolic acidosis is improving.

Circulation

The aim of the fluid replacement is to re-establish Rosie's circulating volume whilst also to remove the ketone bodies from her circulation and correct the electrolyte imbalance. Appropriate fluid replacement is an important initial intervention in DKA, which can help mitigate against a hyperglycaemic internal environment (NICE, 2016). For Rosie, the primary fluid replacement needs to be 0.9% sodium chloride (or 0.9% saline). An initial bolus of 250 mls of 0.9% saline to a maximum of two litres is recommended for her (NICE, 2017a). This should not be infused too rapidly as this can cross the blood brain barrier and result in cerebral oedema.

Rosie needs to be catheterised with a urometer bag in situ. Her urine output should be measured hourly and the input and output recorded on a fluid balance chart with an hourly cumulative balance calculated and a running total maintained. It is advisable to undertake regular urinalysis on Rosie's urine so that the presence of glucosuria can be identified. Potassium replacement is also required early on and Rosie's electrolyte levels should be frequently assessed for the presence of hypokalaemia. This replacement can be premixed with 0/9% sodium chloride dependent on the plasma concentrations (NICE, 2017a).

Disability

Rosie's level of consciousness should be recorded hourly to assess for any decrease in her level of consciousness using APCVU and the GCS.

An intravenous insulin infusion will need to be administered to Rosie. Once her blood glucose level has fallen to 10–15 mmol/l a glucose containing fluid infusion of not more than two litres in 24 hours will then need to be administered. At the same time, she will need a continuous infusion of insulin of around six units/hour to be administered. The insulin is required to clear the ketones and reduce the metabolic acidosis that Rosie is experiencing. The intravenous glucose infusion is to ensure Rosie's blood sugar levels do not drop too low with the insulin infusion (NICE, 2016). Rosie may also need to have a naso-gastric tube inserted and naso-gastric feeding slowly commenced (NICE, 2016), and anti-emetics provided to prevent Rosie from vomiting further.

Exposure

Rosie's pressure areas need to be assessed at all times and if she becomes unable to change her position, she will need help to do so and she may also need to be nursed on a low air loss mattress. Similarly, Rosie will need to undergo a venous thromboembolism (VTE) assessment for the potential of developing a Deep Vein Thrombosis (DVT). Rosie may also need anti-embolic stockings and an injection of heparin based on the results of the assessment. As her oral mucosa and eyes are dry and sore, she will also need regular eyecare with sterile water and mouthcare including brushing with toothpaste and a toothbrush.

Rosie's mother has been with her throughout the admission. She is very anxious and not keen to leave Rosie's bedspace. Her father is at home with Rosie's 12-year-old sister. The family are well known to the local diabetic team in the community and so it is important that Rosie and her mother have access to these specialists for support and advice.

Conclusion

To summarise, Rosie has experienced an acute diabetic emergency in the form of DKA. Due to her Type I diabetes, she has decreased insulin secretion. As her blood glucose level rises, glucose tips into the urine and this draws more fluid out of the circulation to be excreted and Rosie develops polyuria. Consequently, she becomes dehydrated and has a metabolic acidosis not only due to her hypovolaemia and reduced peripheral perfusion, but also due to the breakdown of adipose tissue to release stored form of glucose to increase blood sugar levels further. This results in ketone bodies being secreted, which add to Rosie's metabolic acidosis. Treatment involves sensible fluid resuscitation and insulin therapy.

CASE STUDY 9.4: DELIRIUM – FLORENCE SMITH

Box 9.5 Florence's initial assessment

Florence Smith fell and fractured her femur and has had this surgically repaired. She is an 84-year-old lady recovering from her surgery on a post-operative ward. Florence is a widowed lady who lives on her own and is usually independent, she is a retired bookkeeper and an active member of her local church. After her operation she appeared very confused, disorientated and aggressive at night, trying to pull her cannula out and shouting at the nurses. When her daughter visited during the day, Florence was quiet and sleepy; she was distressed to hear about her mother's behaviour during the night as this was completely out of character.

Florence weighs 70 kg.

Airway

- Florence is able to speak in full sentences

Breathing

- Respiratory rate: 16 breaths per minute (bpm)
- Oxygen saturation levels: 96% on air
- Chest clear on examination

Circulation

- Blood pressure: 140/80 mmHg
- Heart rate: 85 beats per minute, Sinus Rhythm
- Temperature: 37.2°C
- Urine output not measured
- Capillary refill time (CRT): 1 second

Disability

- Confused on ACVPU at night, recorded as alert during day
- Pain score 1/3, receiving regular post-operative analgesia
- Blood glucose: 6.0 mmol/l

Exposure

- Pressure areas intact
- Skin well perfused

Case study 9.4 looks at a patient with delirium. During the course of your studies, and even through reading this book, you will have become familiar with the terms *cardiovascular failure* and *respiratory failure*, but how familiar are you with the term 'acute brain failure'? Page and Ely (2015) suggest that we should think of the term 'delirium' as an acute organ failure, maybe then it will have the prominence in nursing and medical care that it deserves. For some healthcare practitioners, a period of acute confusion, paranoia and restlessness can be seen as an inevitable consequence of a stay in an acute hospital environment; however for a patient, their family and friends, this is entirely unexpected, scary and frightening.

Delirium (sometimes called an 'acute confusional state') is a common clinical syndrome characterised by disturbed consciousness, cognitive function or perception (NICE, 2010, updated 2019). It is a serious condition that is associated with poor outcomes; however it can be prevented and if recognised early can be treated. The Latin *deliro-delirare* means 'going off track' with the term 'ICU psychosis' previously used to describe the condition. However, delirium is not solely confined to the ICU environment; key high-risk groups identify its prevalence in all areas with a recent focus on also identifying delirium in the community (NICE, 2017b). There are key high-risk groups:

- Age 65 years or older
- Current hip fracture
- Cognitive impairment (past or present) and/or dementia
- Severe illness

Clearly, all the patients we have been considering in this text are at high risk of delirium as they are admitted due to severe illness. Indeed some intensive care unit patients may have as many as ten risk factors for delirium. Page and Ely (2015) identified 61 risk factors in 27 studies for delirium. Delirium is not a description of a behaviour but a medical diagnosis of a syndrome.

Identification of delirium is important because of its association with poorer outcomes for patients and patient safety risks. It is associated with:

- Increased risk of self-extubation and removal of catheters
- Increased hospital stay
- Increased risk of long-term cognitive impairment
- Increased mortality
- Increased incidence of dementia
- Higher incidence of falls and pressure ulcers

Delirium is a common condition, although many studies identify that it is under-recognised (Sikhamoni, 2016; Zamoscik et al., 2017). Prevalence of delirium according to Page and Ely (2015) is:

- 1:6 delirious in any ward
- 1:5 HDU
- 4:5 ventilated patients
- 2:5 acute geriatric ward
- 3:5 fractured neck of femur

There are different types of delirium but in fact most patients will develop a combination of hyper and hypo active delirium (see Table 9.4). Anecdotal experience would indicate that hyperactive is dominant at night and hypoactive during the hours of daylight.

Table 9.4   Types of delirium

Types of delirium
Hyperactive – paranoid, agitated
<ul><li>Readily recognised, best prognosis</li><li>Purely hyperactive: 1.6% of delirium episodes</li><li>Often linked to drug/alcohol withdrawal</li></ul>
Hypoactive – withdrawn, quiet, paranoid
<ul><li>'Quiet' delirium</li><li>Often not well recognised, misdiagnosed</li><li>Purely hypoactive episodes 43.5%</li><li>Linked to metabolic causes and hypoxia</li></ul>
Mixed – combination
<ul><li>Most common 54.9%</li><li>Worst prognosis</li></ul>

Hyperactive forms of delirium affect the smallest number of patients and see an increased number of spontaneous movements, as well as moving more quickly, for example flailing arm, pulling at clothes or lines, shouting out and disorientation.

Hypoactive episodes of delirium see a reduced speed in initiating and continuing movements, both spontaneous and when completing a command. This can result in a patient who is 'still', withdrawn, avoids contact and is disorientated.

Mixed forms of delirium, which are the most common see a fluctuation between hypoactive and hyperactive states.

Pathophysiology of delirium is poorly understood but leading theories attribute this to an imbalance of neurotransmitters, predominantly an excess of dopamine, which controls the brain's reward and pleasure centres, regulates movement and is involved in the emotional response. Other explanations focus on stress hormones triggering an imbalance and the role of inflammation as part of a chronic neurodegenerative change in altering brain function.

This can be compounded in infection or trauma, which may require surgery and add to the present inflammatory state.

Precipitating factors and preventative measures are more widely agreed on (see Table 9.5).

Table 9.5   Precipating Factors and Preventative Measures in Delirium

Precipitating factors	Preventative measures
Surgery	
Dehydration	Adequate hydration
Poor nutrition	Adequate nutrition
Constipation	Address constipation
Infection	Effective use of NEWS2 and qSOFA
Immobility	Early mobilisation
Pain	Effective pain assessment and management
Hypoxia	Effective assessment and management of hypoxaemia
Sleep deprivation	Promote sleep
Neurological disease	Cognitively stimulating activities
Deliriogenic drugs	Review of medication
	Orientation
	Provide clock
	Address hearing and sight impairment
	Family and friends' involvement

Sources: NICE, 2010, updated 2019; Page & Ely, 2015; Shaughnessy, 2013

Keeping patients in touch with reality is a key role for all healthcare professionals in the understanding that family members and friends provide a vital link with the real world to patients. Some areas have changed visiting practice as a result of the recommendations of NICE CG103 (2010, updated 2019), reverting to an open visiting policy so that healthcare professionals can facilitate family participation in care and communicate effectively with them to understand why their loved one is delirious.

Management

Management of delirium in the UK is driven by the clinical driver NICE CG103 *Delirium: prevention, diagnosis and management* (NICE, 2010, updated 2019). This is due for further update of risk assessment and diagnosis.

Assessment

Florence's observations were being carried out four hourly and the NEWS2 (Royal College of Physicians [RCP], 2017) calculated for Florence during the day was 0 and 3 during the night owing to her night-time confusion and disorientation. This score of 0–4 identified a low clinical risk and a ward-based response. The nurse noted that the urine output had not been measured; Florence had a urinary catheter post-operatively but this was removed 24 hours after surgery.

The nurse looking after Florence however recognised that the behaviour demonstrated during the night and sleepiness and withdrawal during the day were potential signs of delirium, which is common in post-operative hip replacement patients. The nurse had listened to Florence's daughters' concerns, documenting these in the patient record in readiness for raising this at the ward round later in the morning.

The post-operative ward uses the Confusion Assessment Method (CAM) tool to assess delirium. The nurse had recently attended a study day addressing risk of delirium in hip fracture patients and felt confident in using the tool. CAM screens for the presence of four clinical features of delirium:

- Acute onset and fluctuating course – Florence had had an acute change in her mental status from the baseline; it fluctuated during the day and night.
- Inattention – Florence had difficulty focusing her attention during the day.
- Disorganised thinking – during the night Florence had been disorientated, confused and aggressive, which was out of character.
- Altered level of consciousness – Florence was hyperalert (vigilant) during the night and lethargic but easily roused during the day.

Florence scored positively for each of the four features.

In line with NICE (2010, updated 2019) guidance, the nurse ensured that Florence was in an easily observable area of the ward and took time to explain to Florence and her daughter any interventions that were undertaken and the plan of care for that day. The nurse ensured that the team knew that Florence should not be moved from this area of the ward. A clock with clear numerals was placed in sight of Florence's bed space and her wrist watch applied; the team caring for Florence were encouraged to include which day of the week it was in conversation, the month, the time and make reference to events outside of the hospital environment to keep her in touch with reality. Florence wore reading glasses and had a hearing aid; these were kept close at hand for application when needed.

The multidisciplinary team involved in Florence's rehabilitation post-operatively and discharge planning encouraged early mobilisation. Effective pain management employed a multimodal approach (see earlier part of this chapter on pain management) so that physiotherapy was more effective.

Regular family visits were encouraged and the family were advised to remind Florence to drink oral fluids to avoid dehydration. Urine output was measured; a catheter was not inserted due to the risk of potential infection and potential to exacerbate Florence's distress. Florence's electrolyte balance was monitored to ensure they remained within normal parameters and a record of bowel movements was made in the notes to detect any risk of constipation.

Florence's family identified that she had a love of music and enjoyed this as part of her church-going. Johnson et al. (2018) identify the benefits of music as an intervention in healthcare settings and particularly the calming effect via neurotransmission from the cerebral cortex through changing levels of cortisol and catecholamines. Post-operative delirium in hip surgery, readiness to ambulate and getting out of bed earlier were positively associated with the use of music intervention. Therefore, Florence's family provided headphones and a device for her to listen to music when not having a family visit during the day.

Florence's medications were reviewed to ensure that they were still required for her safety and wellbeing. Pain was assessed and managed in line with the discussion in Stanley's case study. NICE (2010, updated 2019) guidance recommends the use of short term (1 week or less) haloperidol if verbal or non-verbal techniques to treat distressed people are ineffective or inappropriate. Haloperidol 2–10mg IV was prescribed for Florence as required; this works as a dopamine antagonist in the central nervous system and aids in reducing the frightening perceptual disturbances.

At night, any non-essential interventions were omitted in order to promote sleep and the area kept dark to emphasise the difference between night and day, reducing noise to a minimum.

Conclusion

To conclude, Florence has a combination of hyper and hypoactive delirium following repair of a fractured femur. Florence's age and surgery makes her high risk for developing delirium and she scored positively on all components of the CAM tool. Preventative measures include early mobilization, orientating to place and time, ensuring adequate hydration and nutrition, and family involvement.

Understanding and insight into the experience of delirium for patients is key for healthcare professionals to appreciate. Alongside the patient stories in Page and Ely (2015), there are many online resources and videos that can be utilised.

REFERENCES

Bostock-Cox, B. (2017) Understanding the link between obesity and diabetes. *Nursing Standard*, 31 (44), 52–62.

Bulger, E. M., Arneson, M A., Mock, C. N. & Jurkovich, G. J. (2000) Rib fractures in the elderly. *Journal of Trauma*, 48, 1040–1047.

Connolly, E.S., Rabenstein, A. A., Carhuapoma, J. R., Derdeyn, C. P., Dion, J., Higashida, R. T., Hoh, B. L., Kirkness, C. J., Naidech, A. M., Ogilvy, C. S., Patel, A. B., Thompson, B. G., Vespa, P., American Heart Association Stroke Council, Council on Cardiovascular Radiology and Intervention, Council on Cardiovascular Nursing, Council on Cardiovascular Surgery and Anaesthesia & Council on Clinical Cardiology (2012) Guidelines for the management of aneurysmal subarachnoid haemorrhage. *Stroke*, 43 (6), 1711–1737.

Dauri, M., Fabbi, E., Gatti, A., Celidonio, L., Carpenedo, R. & Sabato, A.F. (2009) Gabapentin and Pregabalin for the acute post-operative pain management. A systematic narrative review of the recent clinical evidence. *Current Drug Targets*, 10 (8), 716–733.

Derbyshire, J. & Hill, B. (2018) Performing neurological observations. *British Journal of Nursing*, 27 (19), 1110–1114.

Farsani, F.S., Brodovicz, K., Soleymanlou, N., Marquard, J., Wissinger, E. & Maies, B.A. (2017) Incidence and prevalence of diabetic ketoacidosis (DKA) among adults with type 1 diabetes mellitus (T1D): A systematic literature review. *BMJ Open*, 7 (7).

Gelinas, C., Fillion, L., Puntillo, K., Viens, C. & Fortier, M. (2006) Validation of the critical care pain observation tool in adult patients. *American Journal of Critical Care*, 15 (4), 420–427.

Gosmanov, A. R., Gosmanova, E. O. & Dillard-Cannon, E. (2014) Management of adult diabetic ketoacidosis. *Diabetes, Metabolic Syndrome and Obesity: Targets and Therapy*, 7, 255–264.

Hickey, J. V. & Strayer, A. L. (2019) *The Clinical Practice of Neurological and Neurosurgical Nursing* (8th ed.). Philadelphia: Wolters Kluwer.

Intercollegiate Stroke Working Party (2016) *Sentinel Stroke National Audit Programme acute organisational audit report*. Available at: www.strokeaudit.org/Documents/National/AcuteOrg/2016/2016-AOANationalReport.aspx (accessed 28 January 2022).

Johnson, K., Fleury, J. & McClain, D. (2018) Music intervention to prevent delirium among older patients admitted to a trauma intensive care unit and a trauma orthopaedic unit. *Intensive and Critical Care Nursing*, 47, 7–14.

Lindner, L. M. E., Gontscharuk, V., Bachle, C., Castillo, K., Stahl-Pehe, A., Tonnies, T., Yossa, R., Holl, R. W. & Rosenbauer, J. (2018) Severe hypoglycemia and diabetic ketoacidosis in young persons with preschool onset of type 1 diabetes mellitus: An analysis of three nationwide population-based surveys. *Paediatric Diabetes*, 19 (4), 713–720.

Marcovitch, H. (Ed.) (2010) *Black's Medical Dictionary*. London: A & C Black.

Matthys, J., Elwyn, G., Van Nuland, M., Van Maele, G., De Sutter, A., De Meyere, M. & Deveugele, M. (2009) Patients' ideas, concerns, and expectations (ICE in general practice). *British Journal of General Practice*, January, 29–36.

National Confidential Enquiry into Patient Outcome and Death (NCEPOD) (2013) Subarachnoid haemorrhage: Managing the flow. Available at: www.ncepod.org.uk/2013sah.html (accessed 28 January 2022).

NICE (2010, updated 2019) *Delirium: prevention, diagnosis and management*, CG103. Available at: www.nice.org.uk/guidance/cg103 (accessed 28 January 2022).

NICE (2016) *Type 1 diabetes in adults: Diagnosis and management*, NG17. Available at: www.nice.org.uk/guidance/ng17/ifp/chapter/diabetic-ketoacidosis (accessed 28 January 2022).

NICE (2017a) *Intravenous fluid therapy in adults in hospital*, CG174. Available at: www.nice.org.uk/Guidance/CG174 (accessed 28 January 2022).

NICE (2017b) *Recognising and preventing delirium. A quick guide for care home managers*. Available at: www.nice.org.uk/media/default/about/nice-communities/social-care/quick-guides/delirium-quick-guide-1.pdf (accessed 28 January 2022).

NICE (2019) *Head injury: Assessment and early management*, CG176. Available at: www.nice.org.uk/Guidance/CG176 (accessed 28 January 2022).

Page, V. J. & Ely, E. W. (2015) *Delirium in Critical Care*. Cambridge: Cambridge University Press.

Pasero, C. & McCaffery, M. (2011) *Pain Assessment and Pharmacological Management*. St Louis: Elsevier Mosby.

Resuscitation Council UK (2015) *The ABCDE approach*. Available at: www.resus.org.uk/library/2015-resuscitation-guidelines/abcde-approach (accessed 27 January 2022).

Royal College of Physicians (RCP) (2016) *National clinical guideline for stroke*. Available at: www.strokeaudit.org/SupportFiles/Documents/Guidelines/2016-National-Clinical-Guideline-for-Stroke-5t-(1).aspx (accessed 28 January 2022).

Royal College of Physicians (RCP) (2017) *National Early Warning Score (NEWS) 2*. Available at: www.rcplondon.ac.uk/projects/outputs/national-early-warning-score-news-2 (accessed 28 January 2022).

Sikhamoni, S. (2016) Inspiring colleagues to learn about delirium. *Nursing Standard*, 31 (9), 18–20.

Shaughnessy, L. (2013) Introducing delirium screening in a cardiothoracic critical care unit. *Nursing in Critical Care*, 18 (1), 8–13.

Zamoscik, K., Godbold, R. & Freeman, P. (2017) Intensive care nurses' experiences and perceptions of delirium and delirium care. *Intensive and Critical Care Nursing*, 40, 94–100.

10
EXPOSURE: A CASE STUDY
SARAH MCGLOIN

Chapter learning outcomes

By the end of this chapter you will be able to:

1. Appreciate the difficulties that patients have with the transitions in the level of care they receive.
2. Understand the longer term physiological effects of being acutely unwell.
3. Be aware of the longer term psychosocial aspects of being acutely unwell.
4. Recognise the need for rehabilitation following a period of acute/critical care.

Key words

- Rehabilitation
- Transitional care
- Post-Traumatic Stress Disorder (PTSD)
- Delirium
- Psychosocial aspects of care

INTRODUCTION

This chapter presents a final case study that considers a range of issues as the patient transitions from higher levels of care with more staff to a lower level of care. The longer term physiological effects of an acute illness on a patient's recovery and rehabilitation will be considered as will the range of psychosocial issues experienced by many. The nurse's role in the transition in care will also be explored to support nurses to care for patients moving from higher levels of care.

CASE STUDY 10.1: SURVIVING COVID-19 – TONY WARD

This case study explores the case of Tony Ward. Tony was admitted to the Emergency Department (ED) two days before Easter following a three-day history of flu-like symptoms. Tony had a temperature, a new persistent cough and had lost his sense of taste. Tony had insisted on going to work despite feeling very poorly.

Box 10.1

On a Monday morning, Tony said goodbye to his wife and three daughters and left for work, still feeling quite poorly. As Tony got to his desk, he collapsed. The air ambulance was called and Tony received critical care at the scene. Tony was transferred by air to the local hospital and a quick SOFA score of 3 identified sepsis. The Sepsis Six care bundle was commenced within 20 minutes of his admission to the Emergency Department. A test for COVID-19 came back as positive. Tony was transferred shortly afterwards to the Critical Care Unit (CCU) as he was assessed to be a Level 3 critical care patient (Intensive Care Society, 2021). Tony was managed on the CCU where he remained for three weeks.

Tony was initially intubated and ventilated, but the endotracheal tube was changed for a tracheostomy tube four days following his admission. Tony was nursed in the prone position to aid his ventilation. Tony required cardiovascular support in the form of fluids and vasopressors, he also experienced Acute Kidney Injury and required support from continuous veno-venous haemofiltration for ten days. Tony was a Level 3 critical care patient throughout this period and received sedation. After ten days on sedation, sedation holds at this time identified that he was ready to be weaned from ventilation. Sedation was stopped and slowly Tony's level of consciousness improved.

Gradually, the level of respiratory support was decreased but Tony still needed his tracheostomy and a small amount of Continuous Positive Airway Pressure (CPAP). Although he remained

(Continued)

on the CCU, Tony became a Level 2 critical care patient and a speaking valve helped him communicate with his family. The CPAP was soon weaned off and the decision was taken to remove the tracheostomy. Tony had been sitting out of bed for a couple of hours each day but he still required a urinary catheter and was unable to eat or drink and so received feeding via a nasogastric tube. Tony was discharged to the ward two days after his tracheostomy was removed.

The discharge took place late in the afternoon at teatime as the CCU needed Tony's bed for a new Level 3 critical care patient who had come into the ED as an emergency admission. Just prior to the discharge, Tony still had his blood pressure monitored continually through an arterial line and his heart rate and rhythm were also continuously monitored. Tony had an oxygen saturation probe in place, which continuously monitored his oxygen saturations. He liked to use this as a call bell when he needed a nurse as he knew that when he removed the probe, the monitor would alarm and a nurse would immediately appear. Tony was not able to be visited by his wife and children throughout his hospital stay but communicated with them via the hospitals iPads through FaceTime.

Levels of care

The Comprehensive Critical Care policy (DH, 2000) was that the level of physiological support required by a patient should be determined by their level of dependency and not their geographical location (DH, 2000; Hillman, 2002; ICS, 2021). The guidance within Comprehensive Critical Care (DH, 2000) proposed 'critical care without walls' where critical care should be delivered in a range of settings so as to include emergency care, acute care wards and critical care follow-up services and not just the CCU (DH, 2000; Marshall et al., 2017). To assist practitioners with this model of critical care, the ICS (2021) devised the levels of care framework presented in Table 10.1.

Table 10.1 The levels of care framework as proposed by the UK Intensive Care Society (ICS, 2009, 2021)

Ward Care	Patients whose needs can be met through normal ward care in an acute hospital.
	• Patients who have recently been relocated from a higher level of care, but their needs can be met on an acute ward with additional advice and support from the critical care outreach team.
	• Patients who can be managed on a ward but remain at risk of clinical deterioration.
Level 1 enhanced care	Patients requiring more detailed observations or interventions, including basic support for a single organ system and those 'stepping down' from higher levels of care.
	• Patients requiring interventions to prevent further deterioration or rehabilitation needs that cannot be met on a normal ward.
	• Patients who require ongoing interventions (other than routine follow up) from critical care outreach teams to intervene in deterioration or to support escalation of care.
	• Patients needing a greater degree of observation and monitoring that cannot be safely provided on a ward, judged on the basis of clinical circumstances and ward resources.
	• Patients who would benefit from Enhanced Perioperative Care.

(Continued)

Table 10.1   (Continued)

Level 2 critical care	Patients requiring increased levels of observations or interventions (beyond level 1) including basic support for two or more organ systems and those 'stepping down' from higher levels of care.
	• Patients requiring interventions to prevent further deterioration or rehabilitation needs, beyond that of level 1.
	• Patients needing two or more basic organ system monitoring and support.
	• Patients needing one organ systems monitored and supported at an advanced level (other than advanced respiratory support).
	• Patients needing long term advanced respiratory support.
	• Patients who require level 1 care for organ support but who require enhanced nursing for other reasons, in particular maintaining their safety if severely agitated.
	• Patients needing extended post-operative care, outside that which can be provided in enhanced care units: extended postoperative observation is required either because of the nature of the procedure and/or the patient's condition and co-morbidities.
	• Patients with major uncorrected physiological abnormalities, whose care needs cannot be met elsewhere.
	• Patients requiring nursing and therapies input more frequently than available in level 1 areas.
Level 3 critical care	Patients needing advanced respiratory monitoring and support alone.
	• Patients requiring monitoring and support for two or more organ systems at an advanced level.
	• Patients with chronic impairment of one or more organ systems sufficient to restrict daily activities (co-morbidity) and who require support for an acute reversible failure of another organ system.
	• Patients who experience delirium and agitation in addition to requiring level 2 care.
	• Complex patients requiring support for multiple organ failures, this may not necessarily include advanced respiratory support.

If a patient dependency level progresses from Level 2 to Level 1, they are usually transferred from the CCU to an acute care ward where they continue to receive physical and psychological support (ICS, 2021). Patients are normally then discharged from the ward into the community (the patient's home or a community-based facility) (ICS, 2015). Tony was initially a Level 3 critical care patient, became a Level 2 critical care patient whilst on the CCU and was then transferred as a Level 1 patient to the ward where he became a ward-level patient. He was eventually discharged when his dependency level demonstrated that he was ready to return home.

COVID-19

Tony has been admitted with COVID-19, which is a novel coronavirus first identified in China in late 2019 with the first cases identified in the UK in January 2010. On 11 March 2020, the WHO characterised COVID-19 as a pandemic. The coronavirus is the source of the infection. The main route of transmission is through respiratory droplets and close contact with individuals (WHO, 2020).

Rehabilitation

Tony, like many others who have had COVID-19, became critically ill and spent time on CCU. As such he had many of the symptoms any critical care patient may demonstrate following a critical care stay, including:

- Dyspnoea
- Anxiety
- Depression
- Prolonged pain
- Impaired physical function
- Poor quality of life (QoL) (Denehy & Elliott, 2012; Zhao et al., 2020)

This combination of physical, cognitive and psychological issues is known as post-intensive care syndrome (PICS) (Jackson et al., 2014). Patients who experience PICS require a holistic approach to managing these issues (Zhao et al., 2020).

With COVID-19 being a novel coronavirus, there is limited evidence available for a rehabilitation strategy for patients experiencing the disease. Zeng et al., (2020) have developed a rehabilitation programme based upon the WHO Family of International Classifications (WHO-FICs) framework, which focuses on the diagnosis, then evaluation of the disease in response to the therapeutic interventions. The rehabilitation approach can include preventive, therapeutic, health-promoting and palliative care according to the individual needs of the patient (Qiu et al., 2020). Therapeutic methods are mainly used in hospitals when the patients are inpatients.

According to the NICE (2009) in their guidance *Rehabilitation after critical illness in adults*, rehabilitation should commence at the very beginning of the patient journey starting from the patient's admission, through to ward care and then following discharge. Tony experienced, like many, a dry cough, a temperature and extreme fatigue. He also lost his sense of taste. It took a week for his symptoms to worsen to dyspnoea and hypoxia. His chest X-ray on admission showed bilateral basal consolidation and there was evidence of airway secretions, which were partially obstructing his airway. His arterial blood gases showed a metabolic acidosis and a respiratory rate of 38 breaths per minute. Tony received critical care and at this point his rehabilitation commenced using therapeutic interventions.

It is clear that patients who experience critical illness and have been admitted to critical care can suffer a range of physical and psychosocial problems during their recovery phase. Unfortunately, a significant proportion of these patients never return to their pre-critical care health status (Bench & Day, 2009).

The initial therapeutic interventions that Tony received were aimed at supporting his respiratory and cardiovascular system. However, as his condition improved, the priorities of his rehabilitation shifted.

The initial rehabilitation period

Initially, interventions on the CCU were aimed at supporting Tony's pulmonary and cardiovascular systems in relation to the effects of the COVID-19 virus.

Pulmonary rehabilitation (PR) is a patient-centred therapeutic intervention involving the multidisciplinary team. PR can be defined as:

> a multidisciplinary intervention based on personalised evaluation and treatment which includes, but is not limited to, exercise training, education, and behavioural modification designed to improve the physical and psychological condition of people with respiratory disease. (Spruit et al., 2013: 13)

Tony's initial PR included chest physiotherapy whilst he was on the CCU. Here the physiotherapist used body position drainage, vibration and clapping, and an active cycle of breathing techniques to support his pulmonary function. The aim of these exercises along with humidification of gases was to clear the airway, through loosening secretions and encouraging Tony to cough and expectorate (Zeng et al., 2020). He was encouraged to mobilise early on, initially sitting out of bed and progressing to walking around his bedspace on the CCU with help from the physiotherapist and nurses.

However, as Tony's condition improved, his PR soon progressed to treating the secondary issues that were contributing to his condition rather than his respiratory condition. Previous Severe Acute Respiratory Syndrome (SARS) type infections have demonstrated that an individual's lung function can be mildly to moderately affected. This is due to the muscle weakness some patients can experience as long as two months following discharge. Beyond respiratory function, other studies on previous SARS patients from the 2003 and 2009 epidemics found their cardiorespiratory systems and musculoskeletal performance were also badly affected and these also impacted upon their overall quality of life (Hui et al., 2005; Lau et al., 2005).

CARDIAC REHABILITATION

As well as demonstrating the characteristics of Post Intensive Care Syndrome (PICS), Tony also experienced arrhythmias and damage to his myocardium from the virus itself. Whilst on the CCU he also experienced hypoxia, hypotension and elevated systemic inflammatory response, which are all associated with COVID-19 (Kochi et al., 2020). As such, as his condition improved Tony required cardiac rehabilitation, which aimed for him to return to work in a physically and psychologically fit state thus enhancing his quality of life outcomes (Cowie et al., 2019).

Cardiac rehabilitation (CR) is based upon six core components:

- health behaviour change and education
- lifestyle risk factor management
- psychosocial health

- medical risk management
- long-term strategies, and audit and evaluation.

CR is now recommended in international guidelines, with increasing evidence that CR can improve exercise capacity, QoL outcomes and psychological wellbeing as well as reducing mortality and morbidity rates and further hospital admissions. Whilst formal CR programmes usually begin several weeks or months after a critical care admission, the process actually starts much earlier with education, protection, mobilisation and reassurance (Cowie et al., 2019).

TRANSITIONAL CARE

A patient who has been critically ill like Tony experiences many transitions from the time they are admitted to hospital to the moment they return home (Chaboyer et al, 2005). Transitions in relation to healthcare have been defined quite simply as:

> ... a passage or movement from one state, condition or place, to another. (Schumaker & Meleis, 1994: 119)

Like many patients, when it was time to leave the CCU, Tony found the move to the ward frightening. Tony was concerned that ward nurses would not understand what had happened to him and that he had been so critically ill. He was worried that because of this lack of insight into his time on the critical care unit, they would not be able to provide the level of care he felt he needed. In particular, Tony was scared to lose the one-to-one care he had received on the unit. The biggest issue for Tony when he was on the ward was having to wait for care. He was used to alerting the nurse on the CCU that he needed the commode and they would be there immediately. When he went to the ward he found himself waiting half an hour for a commode and by the time it arrived it was too late.

The transition of care from the critical care unit to the ward is a challenge associated with feelings of high levels of anxiety, fear and a loss of security (Chaboyer, 2005). As in Tony's case there is often a lack of time to prepare patients for the ward. In some hospitals, specialist nurses assist the transition or the critical care outreach teams may visit those patients recently discharged from critical care. In other hospitals, the critical care nurses themselves visit the patients on the ward, but this is often done in their own time during their comfort break.

It has to be said though that not all patients experience difficulties with moving from the CCU to the ward. Some report positive feelings about the transition, describing the pleasure and excitement associated with leaving critical care. They described how they were pleased to be removed from constraints caused by the technical equipment and be able to look forward to the second chance at life critical care had often provided.

It is not just the patients who find the transition in care from critical care to the ward challenging. Ward nurses can feel stressed due to a feeling of lack of control at having to receive a patient from the CCU who they know has been very sick. This anxiety is often made worse by the lack of frequency of use of some of the clinical skills required to care for these patients. Their stress is also added to by an often perceived lack of competence from the patient and relative. These factors give further cause for concern over patient safety at this time (Bench & Day, 2009).

For the patient and their family moving from critical care to the ward, there are three major areas of focus:

1. Their physical response to their illness and the move to the ward.
2. Their psychological response.
3. Their concerns about provision of care. (Strahan & Brown, 2005)

Physiological issues

The main physiological difficulties that patients face when they are discharged to the ward include lethargy, weakness and fatigue, which are associated with a loss of muscle mass. There is also impaired mobility, pain and a loss of appetite (Strahan & Brown, 2005; Field et al., 2008). Patients also experience difficulties with swallowing and eating due to a reduced pulmonary reserve and coughing. They can also be prone to falling due to postural hypotension.

Psychological issues

Psychological responses include a mix of positive and negative feelings and the importance of family presence while healing. Psychologically, patients may suffer high levels of anxiety, sleep disturbances, nightmares, hallucinations, amnesia and symptoms of depression and post-traumatic stress following a stay in critical care (Jones et al., 2003). Some of these symptoms can also be related to transfer anxiety or relocation stress. This can be defined as:

> ... a state in which an individual experiences physio-logic and or psychological disturbances as a result of transfer from one environment to another (Carpenito, 1993: 728).

What is clear is that all healthcare workers are responsible to recognise and minimise the effects of transfer anxiety and the negative impact it can have on the recovery of a patient such as Tony. However, nurses are in an ideal position to make patient transfers a more positive experience.

> Josephine was the nurse on the ward due to admit Tony from critical care. She recalls:
>
> I started my shift with the Sister informing me, 'Josephine, you're going to get another patient from the critical care. His name is Tony Ward. Apart from that I know nothing about him. Give critical care a call for a handover'. I had previous experiences with patients who were transferring out of critical care units and into my area. I wondered how this patient and family would react to the move to my ward.
>
> Josephine called the critical care unit and spoke to the nurse in charge of the unit that day, Doreen.

The main goal during a patient handover from critical care to the ward is to ensure optimal patient care and safety. Improving team communication can be an important factor in creating patient safety. Both the nurse giving information (Doreen) and the nurse receiving information (Josephine) need to feel comfortable about the communication. Important information regarding the patient plan of care may be missed without effective communication between staff members. There are a number of issues associated with patient transfers from critical care to the ward. These include:

- Physical responses.
- Psychological responses, information and communication.
- Safety and security.
- The needs of relatives (Cullinane & Plowright, 2013).

THE HANDOVER BETWEEN CRITICAL CARE AND THE WARD

> Josephine recalled:
>
> As I received the handover from the critical care nurse, Doreen, via the telephone, I did not have a clear picture of Mr Ward. Doreen was interrupted multiple times with pressing matters from the staff on critical care as she was in charge of the shift that day. I therefore had to admit Tony without a complete history or handover.

This scenario is all too frequent and can add stress to the nurses on both ends of the patient transfer. In this case, Doreen, the nurse transferring the patient out of critical care, as well as Josephine, the receiving nurse, feel rushed and stressed. It is essential that Josephine, as the ward nurse, reassures Tony and his family, keeping in mind his dependency level and needs.

> An added issue with Tony's discharge was that because of the situation in relation to COVID-19, his family were unable to visit him in hospital. This was causing them a great deal of distress and they were constantly on the telephone. Consequently, Josephine had the challenging task of educating Tony and his family of the differences between the critical care unit and the ward.

In the meantime, Doreen was under pressure to discharge Tony to the ward from members of the multidisciplinary team.

> 'Doreen, have you phoned the ward yet about Tony?' demanded the consultant in charge of Critical Care, 'we need to get the patient out of recovery in 20 minutes', she continued. Yes, Doreen had handed over, but she's not sure how clear that was to Josephine. Doreen thought that she would be able to clear up any problems when she got to the ward.
> 'Tony, we need to pack up your belongings because you are moving to another ward', Doreen explained to Tony. She explained that he would be able to get more rest on the ward. Doreen was not sure that Tony and his family felt the same way.

RELOCATION STRESS

Relocation stress can be exacerbated by critical care patients' often poor memory. They often have a limited memory of their stay in the critical care unit (Paul et al., 2004). They may have even forgotten information that they received regarding the transfer. Information should be presented to the patient in a manner that aims to increase comprehension of the transfer purpose. Information may need to be repeated or given in the form of a discussion so that the patient can take an active role in his or her care. Educational materials should be patient focused to ensure optimal understanding. Unfortunately for Tony, because this transfer took place rapidly at teatime, he had no time to prepare himself mentally for the move and also failed to receive any written information. The issues were exacerbated by the fact that Tony's family were unable to visit and it is known that family presence can help patients' transition from Level 3 care to the ward care (Chaboyer, 2005).

One of the first things Josephine needed to do was explain to Tony and his family (via the telephone) the differences between the CCU and the ward. These included:

- Staffing levels.
- Visiting hours (when visiting is allowed again following COVID-19).

- Layout of the ward.
- How to call for help.
- Waiting rooms.
- Meal times.

Patients should be informed about the differences between the critical care area and the ward. Aspects that need to be identified to the patient and family are changes in staff, policies and procedures. Continuity of care should be paramount when transferring a patient out of critical care. Here, as in many cases, Tony has become accustomed to the critical care staff and has mixed feelings about new staff. Therefore, support during the transition phase for the patient needs to be a high priority. The factors that may increase relocation stress are:

- Change in nurse-to-patient staffing ratio.
- Decrease in monitoring equipment.
- Lack of planning the transfer with the patient.

> As Doreen expected, Tony's family were not happy that he was being transferred to the ward.
>   'Is it really necessary to move him now?', Jenny, Tony's wife, asked Doreen. 'It's really late and he's tired and upset.'
>   Doreen explained the benefits of a transfer to Jenny and that as he was getting much better, he did not need critical care any more. Doreen tried to reassure Tony and his family that this transfer was essential and identified the benefits of the transfer to his recovery.

The critical care nurse is pivotal in easing the patient's and family's anxieties and fears when leaving the critical care area.

Families of critically ill patients also need information. Their understanding of issues revolves around information that is given to them. Families really appreciate communication about processes and plans. This helps them to understand the patient's condition and progress. At the point of transfer out of critical care to the ward, it is the critical care nurse who plays an essential role in disseminating information to the family and they must be knowledgeable and sensitive to family needs to provide continuity of care. The family may have a decreased ability to cope with the stress of having a critically ill loved one, and a transfer can lead to uncertainty and anxiety. However, when on the ward, the ward nurse takes over this communication.

Critical care nurses like Doreen are responsible for helping families to understand the progress that has been made by the patient. A successful transfer between CCU and the ward is based upon effective patient preparation for a transfer and should include education and reiteration of the progress made by the patient. As Doreen aimed to do with her communication with

Tony and his family, the nurse can indicate progress that has been made by the patient and that the condition of the patient has improved. Transferring out of the critical care area should be presented to the patient and family as a positive step in the recovery process. In addition, the nurse can discuss plans with the patient and family to further decrease anxiety.

As Tony moved to the ward, Doreen gathered up the necessary equipment that Tony would need on the ward such as a humidifier for his oxygen therapy. She had ensured that a low air loss mattress was in place and that the ward had a pump for Tony's NG Feed.

On arrival to the ward, Josephine oriented Tony and his family to the policies and procedures of the unit and asked if there were any questions. She was confident that Tony was well informed about the reasons for the transfer and seemed comfortable with the ward. She asked Doreen a few clarification questions regarding the handover. Josephine then thanked Doreen for her help and preparation of Tony and his family and felt secure with the complete nurse-to-nurse handover.

STRATEGIES THAT CAN ENHANCE A TRANSFER FROM CRITICAL CARE TO THE WARD

Written material

Written material aims to educate the patient and family and to decrease the stress associated with a transition to a new location and new staff. One approach makes use of an evidence-based booklet for patients and families getting ready for a transfer out of a critical care unit. Paul et al. (2004) designed and implemented an informational booklet based upon the results of a study that identified the educational needs of patients and families. Results indicated that the patient's and family members' satisfaction with the transfer out of the critical care unit was enhanced when the booklet was provided to them. They could refer to the booklet and more readily retain information. The charity ICU Steps have developed a similar booklet.

To enhance patient transition out of critical care, an informational brochure has also been used. The aim of this brochure was the development of guidelines for critical care nurses during communication with family members about the transfer. The responses from the family members indicated that important issues were the name of the doctor, location and telephone number of the new hospital unit, visiting hours, and nurse-to-patient ratio. Most found the brochure useful to aid a family during the transition from the CCU to the ward.

Standardised reporting methods

Another way to enhance patient transfers is the use of a universal and structured method to handover patient information. The situation-background-assessment-recommendation (SBAR) tool can provide a useful structure for this (Zimmermann, 2006). The SBAR method was originally developed for military use, and for use in communication between nurses and medical colleagues. This method has now been adapted and can be used for a nurse-to-nurse handover. When using SBAR, the current condition of the patient is discussed first, then the background and history. The next section is the physical assessment of the patient and, finally, recommendations and outstanding issues that may need to be addressed now that Tony is on the ward. This provides a well-known systematic method for nurses to report information to decrease confusion. Nurses using the SBAR method feel better prepared with important patient information needed to communicate issues relating to a patient.

Ward follow-up

Another method to ease a transfer out of the critical care unit is through the use of a liaison nurse, often referred to as a 'follow-up' nurse. This nurse can help the patient and their family throughout the transfer process to ease the transition. Some organisations have used the role of the liaison nurse to ease transfer anxiety and relocation stress, as a method to increase continuity of care. Others use their critical care outreach team to fulfil this function. This role could be adopted to facilitate the transfer of patients out of critical care. This nurse can also communicate effectively with other members of the multidisciplinary team regarding pertinent patient information.

Care conferences

Care conferences are another way to help the transfer process. Additional research has been conducted with families of patients admitted to the neuroscience intensive care unit. One group participated in a care conference and a period of introductions to make the families at ease with the idea of a transfer. The conference included an explanation to the family regarding the layout and expectations of the ward to which their loved one would be transferred, as well as the patient's progress and a rehabilitation plan. Another part of the conference revolved around patient-centred goal for the family to work toward. Having a care conference was seen to significantly reduce anxiety in the family members after the transfer.

Time of transfer

An aspect that can determine the ease of transfer is the time of day when the transfer takes place. Daytime transfers allow the patient to see the surroundings and meet the staff. If patients are transferred at night, there are fewer staff available and the patient is in a dark, unfamiliar room, which can result in increased stress and anxiety. During this situation, an appropriate option may be to encourage the patient to contact a family member to decrease anxiety of the transfer.

Post intensive care syndrome

Following his critical care stay, Tony, like many others, experienced post intensive care syndrome (PICS). This is the term given to those critical care survivors who experience new or worsening impairments in physical, cognitive, or mental health that persist beyond their acute hospital admission. PICS causes an impact on the patient's cognitive, physical, and mental wellbeing (Needham et al., 2012). These issues persist beyond CCU for as long as 5–15 years. The major risk factors for the development of PICS are acute respiratory distress syndrome (ARDS), sepsis, delirium, prolonged mechanical ventilation and multiorgan failure. As such, the COVID-19 pandemic will likely result in more patients like Tony experiencing PICS and its associated health and economic challenges.

Screening and assessment tools used in hospital, at discharge, and following discharge should help identify those who would benefit from services and strategies to improve PICS outcomes for patients and their families.

Post intensive care syndrome involves three domains including:

- Post-ICU related weakness
- Prolonged pain
- Psychological and cognitive issues (Denehy & Elliott, 2012; Jackson et al., 2014)

Post critical care weakness rehabilitation

Physical impairment in patients due to PICS is seen in up to 80% of patients and includes muscular weakness, fatigue, dyspnoea, impaired pulmonary function, decreased exercise tolerance, sexual dysfunction and respiratory failure. These all lead to a reduction in activities of daily living and quality of life (Needham et al., 2012).

It is not yet clear how COVID-19 affects survivors' musculoskeletal system (Barker-Davies et al., 2020). However, patients who have been admitted to CCU during previous SARS epidemics have suffered musculoskeletal complications that have required rehabilitation. Tony, like many others, received early mobilisation within the CCU where it has been shown to be practical and safe (Connolly et al., 2016). Tony was assisted initially to sit out of bed even whilst he received haemofiltration and progressed to walking around his bedspace on the CU prior to discharge to the ward.

As with many critical care patients who have received mechanical ventilation, Tony experienced weakness and physical impairments not directly attributable to his COVID-19 (Appleton et al., 2015). It is well known that a period of prolonged mechanical ventilation and immobilisation results in musculoskeletal changes. The 'critical care acquired weakness' Tony experienced following his CCU stay included critical illness associated polyneuropathy, myopathy and neuromyopathy (Appleton et al., 2015). He also complained of prolonged pain, weakness and dyspnoea. He had lost a significant amount of weight, which was described by his medical team as 'muscle wasting'. In fact it was so bad that some of his acquaintances did not recognise him when he was out and about at home following his discharge.

Because of his prolonged pain, Tony not only received rehabilitation from a musculoskeletal aspect but also from a multidisciplinary pain team, who considered that the musculoskeletal issues went hand in hand with his experiences of pain.

Upon discharge home, Tony's rehabilitation moved to being preventive with health-promotion methods implemented as well as outpatient care for those in the community. Rehabilitation doctors and therapists should develop individualised rehabilitation programmes according to the actual health condition and functional state, the expected outcomes, the expectations of patients and their families, and the actual service's setting (Jones et al., 2003).

COGNITIVE IMPAIRMENT ASSOCIATED WITH PICS

PICS cognitive impairment is noted in 30% to 80% of patients and includes memory loss and difficulty with concentration, comprehension and critical thinking (Colbenson et al., 2019).

These impairments include anxiety, depression and PTSD in patients as well as their carers. As critical care mortality rates improve and critical care survival rates increase (Lilly et al., 2017), healthcare practitioners are now beginning to appreciate the impact that a critical care stay can have on an individual's emotional wellbeing and survivorship long after they leave the critical care unit (Allum et al., 2017). As a result, concerns about long-term outcomes and quality of life – which is packaged under the phrase 'survivorship' – in critical care survivors have become a priority. Recently, more attention has been given to the psychiatric consequences of acute illness in the CCU, especially in younger patients. Psychiatric disorders, including anxiety, depression and PTSD have a strong impact on the survivorship and quality of life in long-term critical care survivors (Jackson et al., 2014).

A clear issue is the deficit in mental health support after hospital discharge for former critical care patients because the focus has always been on physical recovery (Heydon et al., 2020). However, the impact of psychologists or use of psychotherapy in critical care settings is unclear. It is possible that involvement of mental health services whilst in hospital might lead to a more reliable involvement of these services in the community. There is also increasing evidence to suggest that the early use of psychotherapy in the CCU and interventions including patient diaries can lead to improved recovery and outcomes for critical illness survivors. Owing to a potential lack of availability of formally trained psychologists, critical care nurses find themselves becoming the providers of psychotherapy whilst patients are in CCU. This early instigation of therapy to prevent PICS, or to reduce its impact once it has developed, may prove beneficial for CCU and COVID-19 survivors like Tony.

PICS AND COVID-19

Patients like Tony who have experienced severe COVID-19 often develop critical illness with an Acute Respiratory Distress Syndrome (ARDS) presentation (Centers for Disease Control and Prevention, 2021). Patients with COVID-19 treated in the CCU may be at higher risk for developing PICS due to reduced visits from family and friends, prolonged mechanical ventilation, high levels of sedation, and limited physical therapy during and after hospitalization due to social distancing. Post-CCU care for patients in critical care follow-up clinics is also subject to service limitations due to social distancing and limited personal protective equipment. It is expected that not only will rehabilitation needs increase with COVID-19, but there will likely be higher rates of PTSD, depression and substance abuse for patients, families and healthcare workers, which is something that has been seen in large scale disasters before (DePierro et al., 2020).

It is crucial that patients with a critical illness such as COVID-19 are evaluated for the extent of physical, emotional and cognitive impairments with ongoing assessment of their need for physical and occupational therapy, including signs of anxiety, depression, PTSD or cognitive difficulties. It is vital to utilise the ABCDEF bundle (daily assessment of pain, analgesia, sedation, liberation from mechanical ventilation, delirium, mobility, and family engagement) (Marra et al., 2017).

Those patients recovering from COVID-19 have two phases of the disease that have implications for their rehabilitation. As has already been discussed, in the initial acute respiratory phase, early pulmonary rehabilitation is recommended. The prolonged bedrest, immobilisation phase, warrants attention to neuromotor rehabilitation very much like that given to patients requiring acute stroke rehabilitation (Brugliera et al., 2020). This is especially true for older patients, those who are obese or have co-morbidities, or organ failure. Those who have been on critical care for longer than three weeks are most likely to experience PICS.

Whilst Tony was on the CCU, he felt he was experiencing an altered sense of reality. He described these as being dreams, nightmares and hallucinations. The difficulty with these experiences and memories was that Tony was unable to distinguish between what were and were not real events. Tony described this altered sense of reality continuing when he was on the ward. Here he remembered seeing his father who had died three years earlier, sat next to him explaining that everything was going to be fine. Whilst he felt it comforting that his father was reassuring him, he also felt it confusing as he knew that his father was dead.

Tony also described dreams he had whilst he was on the CCU. He described how when the sedation was reduced, he woke up and saw a face in front of him. He saw this to be a nurse. The face seemed anxious and concerned and following that he was re-sedated. Tony explained however, that once the sedation had been reapplied, the face of the nurse became the focus of nightmares he had.

Once he was awake Tony described how he felt the nurse was trying to kill him. He described becoming combative towards the nurse because he did not want her to harm him. This was demonstrated through Tony becoming restless and aggressive and poorly compliant with his treatment whilst in the CCU. He pulled at his lines and in particular pulled his NG tube out all the time.

There were times however when Tony became withdrawn. He seemed disinterested in anything. He would sit passively not interacting with his family and appearing quite withdrawn.

Delirium

The issues relating to delirium are discussed in Chapter 9. However, in an instance such as Tony's, it is essential that the acute care nurse recognises that a patient's behaviour may be the result of delirium. There should be a high level of suspicion of delirium if a patient has recently been discharged from CCU and is appearing agitated and aggressive. At this point it may be helpful to assess for the presence of delirium using the CAM-ICU tool. Additionally, listen to the family. If they are telling you that this is not normal behaviour for their relative, then this should also trigger a high index of suspicion that the patient is experiencing delirium. If the patient is also passive and not really engaged with their care or recovery, this may also be an indication of delirium. Strategies such as re-orientation, promoting an environment that delineates between day and night, mobilising the patient and possible pharmacological intervention with haloperidol may be required to help manage this delirium.

Tony was finally discharged home a few days later. He commented that even though he had a whirlwind of a hospital stay, he understood what was occurring and felt that the staff took ample time to explain everything to him. He believed that this resulted in increased comfort and a positive experience.

Symptoms experienced following discharge home

The main symptoms currently experienced following discharge home by those like Tony who have had COVID-19 and required critical care are:

- Extremely high levels of fatigue.
- New or worsened breathlessness.
- PTSD symptoms were reported by a much higher proportion of females.
- PTSD (more prevalent in younger females than males).
- Symptoms relating to communication, swallow, voice and persistent coughing.
- Mobility and selfcare issues. (Halpin et al., 2020)

POST-TRAUMATIC STRESS DISORDER (PTSD)

PTSD occurs in some individuals when they develop unpleasant memories following a life-threatening or perceived life-threatening event. The individual experiencing PTSD will also experience hyperarousal symptoms and avoidant behaviour related to the traumatic event (APA, 2013). PTSD is also associated with negative changes in cognition and mood. PTSD is traditionally associated with a reaction to warfare or natural disasters but also now includes a reaction to road traffic accidents, sexual assaults and medical conditions such as a critical care admission (Javidi & Yadollahie, 2012).

FOLLOW-UP

Enhancing survivorship, or the quality of survival, is now central to the management of critically ill patients. The NICE Guidelines (CG83) *Rehabilitation after critical illness* (2009) states the need for a structured rehabilitation programme to commence as early as clinically possible once a patient has been discharged from the critical care unit. This should include an individualised, structured rehabilitation programme that addresses both the physical and psychological needs of the patient. This is further supported by the *Guidelines for the Provision of Intensive Care Services* (GPICS) (FICM, 2019), which recommends that critical care units provide multi-professional, interdisciplinary rehabilitation that is co-ordinated across the recovery continuum to optimise patient outcome.

According to Elliott (2016), critical care follow-up should include:

- Clinical decision making in assessing a patient's suitability for commencing/progressing rehabilitation with a critical care patient.
- An appropriate risk assessment.

- A comprehensive physical and non-physical assessment.
- Options of rehabilitation interventions and approaches.
- The identification of adverse events and potential cessation of the intervention.
- Time points of certain actions during the patient pathway, standards that should be met.
- Promotion of increased adherence to rehabilitation programmes by all members of the critical care team.
- Patient-centred care.
- Promotion to include families within the rehabilitation pathway.
- Promote adherence to NICE Guidelines CG83.

Tony undertook an eight-week structured critical care follow-up programme based at his local hospital. This focused on working to develop his physical strength, whilst also providing counselling for him to explore what had happened to him and why he was feeling as he did. The use of a dairy that had been kept by his family members and the staff in critical care helped with this. There was an opportunity for him to revisit his bed-space on the unit. He found this really helpful as it helped him to make sense of his memories of this time, which he found distorted and confusing. His family were also encouraged to attend some of the sessions with him so that they could talk about their experiences, thoughts and feelings too. Tony also received peer support at these sessions as he undertook the gym work with fellow COVID-19 survivors and he found joining a support group, ICU-Steps, really positive. At the end of the programme, Tony described how he felt much stronger both physically and emotionally. Most importantly, Tony felt with all the support he received when he was discharged home, that he had reached a state of closure on this period of his life. Tony was then excited to be able to progress to the second chance of life that critical care had given to him after contracting COVID-19.

REFERENCES

Allum, L., Connolly, B. & McKeown, E. (2017) Meeting the needs of critical care patients after discharge home: A qualitative exploratory study of patients' perspective. *Nursing in Critical Care*, 23 (6), 316–323. doi:10.1111/nicc.12305.

American Psychiatric Association (APA) (2013) *Diagnostic and Statistical Manual of Mental Disorders* (5th ed.). Arlington: American Psychiatric Publishing, Inc.

Appleton, R. T., Kinsella, J. & Quasim, T. (2015) The incidence of intensive care unit-acquired weakness syndromes: A systematic review. *Journal of Intensive Care Society*, 16, 126–136.

Bench, S.D., Day, T.L. and Griffiths, P. (2010) The user experience of critical care discharge: A meta-synthesis of qualitative research. *International Journal of Nursing Studies*. 47 (4), 487–499.

Brugliera, L., Spina, A., Castellazzi, P., Cimino, P., Tettamanti, A., Houdayer, E., Arcuri, P., Alemanno, F., Mortini, P. & Iannaccone, S. (2020) Rehabilitation of COVID-19 patients. *Journal of Rehabilitation Medicine*, 52 (4). doi:10.2340/16501977-267.

Carpenito, L.J. (1993) *Nursing Diagnosis: Application to Clinical Practice* (5th ed.). Philadelphia: Lippincott Williams & Wilkins.

Centers for Disease Control and Prevention (2021) *Interim clinical guidance for management of patients with confirmed coronavirus disease (COVID-19). Available at*: www.cdc.gov/coronavirus/2019-ncov/hcp/clinical-guidance-management-patients.html (accessed 28 January 2022).

Chaboyer, W., Kendall, E., Kendall, M. and Foster, M. (2005) Transfer out of intensive care: a qualitative exploration of patient and family perceptions. *Australian Critical Care*. 18 (4) 138–145

Colbenson, G. A., Johnson, A. and Wilson, M. E. (2019) Post-intensive care syndrome: Impact, prevention, and management. *Breathe* (Sheff), 15 (2), 98–101.

Connolly, B., Salisbury, L. & O'Neill, B. (2016) Exercise rehabilitation following intensive care unit discharge for recovery from critical illness: Executive summary of a Cochrane collaboration systematic review. *Journal of Cachexia, Sarcopenia and Muscle*, 7, 520–526.

Cowie, A., Buckley J. & Doherty, P. (2019) Standards and core components for cardiovascular disease prevention and rehabilitation. *Heart*, 105, 510–515.

Cullinane, J. P. & Plowright, C.I. (2013) Patients' and relatives' experiences of transfer from intensive care unit to wards. *Nursing in Critical Care*, 18 (6), 289–296.

Denehy, L. & Elliott, D. (2012) Strategies for post ICU rehabilitation. *Current Opinion in Critical Care*, 18, 503–508.

Department of Health (2000) Comprehensive critical care: a review of adult critical care services. London: Department of Health.

DePierro, J., Lowe, S. & Katz, C. (2020) Lessons learned from 9/11: Mental health perspectives on the COVID-19 pandemic. *Psychiatry Research*, 288, 113024. doi:10.1016/j.psychres.2020.113024.

Elliott, S. (2016) Development of critical care rehabilitation guidelines in clinical practice: A quality improvement project. *Physiotherapy*, 102, 69–70.

Faculty of Intensive Care Medicine (2019) *Guidelines for the Provision of Intensive Care Services*. London. FICM.

Field, K., Prinjha, S. and Rowan, K. (2008) 'One patient amongst many.': a qualitative analysis of intensive care unit patients' experiences of transferring to the general ward. *Critical Care*. 12 (1) 2–9.

Halpin, S. J., McIvor, C., Wyatt, G., Adams, A., Harvey, O., Mclean, L., Walshaw, C., Kemp, S., Corrado, J., Singh, R., Collins, T., O'Connor, R. J. & Sivan, M. (2020) Post-discharge symptoms and rehabilitation needs in survivors of COVID-19 infection: A cross-sectional evaluation. *Journal of Medical Virology*, 20, 1–10.

Heydon, E., Wibrow, B., Jacques, A., Sonawane, R. & Anstey, M. (2020) The needs of patients with post intensive care syndrome: A prospective, observational study. *Australian Critical Care*, 33, 116–122.

Hillman, K. (2002) Critical care without walls. *Current Opinion in Critical Care*. 8 (6) 594–599.

Hui, D. S., Wong, K. T., Ko, F. W., Tam, L. S., Chan, D. P., Woo, J. & Sung, J. J. (2005) The 1-year impact of severe acute respiratory syndrome on pulmonary function, exercise capacity, and quality of life in a cohort of survivors. *Chest*, 128, 2247–2261.

Intensive Care Society (2021) *Levels of Adult Critical Care Second Edition Consensus Statement*. London. Intensive Care Society.

Jackson, J. C., Pandharipande, P. P., Girard, T. D., Brummel, N. E., Thompson, J. L., Hughes, C. G., Pun, B. T., Vasilevskis, E. E., Morandi, A., Shintani, A. K., Hopkins, R. O., Bernard, G. R., Dittus, R. S. & Ely, E. W. (2014) Depression, post-traumatic stress disorder, and functional disability in survivors of critical illness in the BRAIN-ICU study: A longitudinal cohort study. *Lancet Respiratory Medicine*, 2, 369–379.

Javidi, H. & Yadollahie, M. (2012) Post-traumatic stress disorder. *International Journal of Occupational and Environmental Medicine*, 3, 2–9.

Jones, C., Skirrow, P., Griffiths, R. D., Humphris, G. H., Ingleby, S., Eddleston, J., Waldmann., C. & Gager, M. (2003) Rehabilitation after critical illness: A randomized, controlled trial. *Critical Care Medicine*, 31 (10), 2456–2461.

Kochi, A. N., Tagliari, A. P., Forleo, G. B., Fassini, G. M. & Tondo, C. (2020) Cardiac and arrhythmic complications in patients with COVID-19. *Journal of Cardiovascular Electrophysiology*, 31,1003–1008.

Lau, H. M.-C., Lee, E. W.-C., Wong, C. N.-C., Ng, G. Y., Jones, A. Y. & Hui, D. S. (2005) The impact of severe acute respiratory syndrome on the physical profile and quality of life. *Archives of Physical Medicine and Rehabilitation*, 86, 1134–1140.

Lilly, C. M., Swami, S., Liu, X., Riker, R. R. & Badawi, O. (2017) Five-year trends of critical care practice and outcomes. *Chest*, 152, 723–735.

Marra, A., Ely, E. W., Pandharipande, P. P. & Patel, M. B. (2017) The ABCDEF bundle in critical care. *Critical Care Clinics*, 33 (2), 225–243.

Marshall, J.C., Bosco, L., Adhikari, N.K., Connolly, B., Diaz, J. Dorman, T., Fowler, R., Meyfroidt, G., Nakagawa, S., Pelosi, P., Vincent, J.L., Vollman,. K. and Zimmerman, J. (2017) What is an intensive care unit? A report of the task force of the World Federation of Societies of Intensive and Critical Care Medicine. *Journal of Critical Care*. 37, 270–276.

Needham, D. M., Davidson, J., Cohen, H., Hopkins, R. O., Weinert, C., Wunsch, H., Zawistowski, C., Bemis-Dougherty, A., Berney, S. C., Bienvenu, O. J., Brady, S. L., Brodsky, M. B., Denehy, L., Elliott, D., Flatley, C., Harabin, A. L., Jones, C., Louis, D., Meltzer, W., Muldoon, S. R., Palmer, J. B., Perme, C., Robinson, M., Schmidt, D. M., Scruth, E., Spill, G. R., Storey, C. P., Render, M., Votto, J. & Harvey, M.A. (2012) Improving long-term outcomes after discharge from intensive care unit: Report from a stakeholders' conference. *Critical Care Medicine*, 40 (2), 502–509.

NICE (2009) *Rehabilitation after Critical Illness in Adults*. London: NICE.

Paul, F., Hendry, C. & Cabrelli, L. (2004) Meeting patient and relatives' information needs upon transfer from an intensive care unit: The development and evaluation of an information booklet. *Journal of Clinical Nursing*, 13 (3), 396–405.

Qiu, Z.-Y.., Li, L. & Chen, D. (2020) Research on rehabilitation guidelines using World Health Organization Family International Classifications: Framework and approaches. *Chinese Journal of Rehabilitation Theory and Practice*, 26 (2), 125–135.

Spruit, M. A., Singh, S.J., Garvey, C., et al. (2013) An official American thoracic Society/European Respiratory Society statement: Key concepts and advances in pulmonary rehabilitation. *American Journal of Respiratory and Critical Care Medicine*, 188, 13–64.

Strahan, E.H.E., and Brown, R.J. (2005) A qualitative study of the experiences of patients following transfer from intensive care. *Intensive and Critical Care Nursing*, 21 (3), 160–171.

World Health Organization (WHO) (2020) *Report of the WHO–China Joint Mission on Coronavirus Disease 2019 (COVID-19)*, 16–24 February 2020. Geneva: World Health Organization.

Zeng, B., Chen, D., Qiu, Z., Zhang, M. & Wang, G. (2020) *Expert consensus on protocol of rehabilitation for COVID-19 patients using framework and approaches of WHO International Family Classifications*. Available at: https://onlinelibrary.wiley.com/doi/pdf/10.1002/agm2.12120 (accessed 28 January 2022).

Zhao, H.-M., Xie, Y.-X. & Wang, C. (2020) Recommendations for respiratory rehabilitation in adults with COVID-19. *Chinese Medical Journal*, 133 (13), 1595–1602.

Zimmermann, P. G. (2006) Cutting-edge discussions of management, policy, and program issues in emergency care. *Journal of Emergency Nursing*, 32 (3), 267–273.

11
LAW, ETHICS AND NON-TECHNICAL SKILLS

PATRICIA MACNAMARA, AMANDA YOUNG

Chapter learning outcomes

By the end of this chapter you will be able to:

1. Discuss the legal and ethical contexts in which care is given.
2. Examine the principles of the Mental Capacity Act.
3. Explore the implications of Advance Decisions to Refuse Treatment/Advance Directives (ADRT/AD).
4. Be able to explain Lasting Power of Attorney and its relation to healthcare practice.
5. Discuss Do Not Attempt Cardiopulmonary Resuscitation decisions.
6. Explore palliative and end of life care in acute care.

Key words

- Ethical principles
- Mental capacity
- Consent
- Advanced directive
- Do Not Attempt Cardiopulmonary Resuscitation
- Palliative care

INTRODUCTION

Those of us involved in healthcare are 'in the business of making things better' (Gawande, 2007). In order to meet the challenges of caring for the acutely ill, clinical competence is crucial, but this is not the only challenge facing us. The professional expectations of a nurse are set out in *The Code: Professional Standards of Practice and Behaviour for Nurses and Midwives* (NMC, 2018) and in the 6Cs (Cummings & Bennett, 2012).

Ethics is the discipline whereby we can think about and discuss what constitutes a good life for humans (Crisp, 2014). Aristotle also considered that ethics was a practical discipline; in other words our deliberations should be translated into actions both as individuals and as societies. The institutions a society develops shows what it values and in our society that has meant the development of the National Health Service (NHS). The law also reflects the values of a society: 'It would not be correct to say that every moral obligation involves a legal duty; but every legal duty is founded on a moral obligation' (*R v. Instan* [1893]).

This chapter will explore how the law upholds the values of our society in relation to healthcare and the obligations this imposes on healthcare professionals. It is worth noting that the law rarely distinguishes between the various healthcare disciples. It is usually interested in competence rather than qualifications. When, for example, the word 'doctor' is used, any other healthcare profession can be substituted:

> .... a wider range of healthcare professionals now provide treatment and advice of one kind or another to members of the public, either as individuals, or as members of a team drawn from different professional backgrounds with the consequence that, although this judgment is concerned particularly with doctors, it is also relevant, *mutatis mutandis*, to other healthcare providers (Montgomery v Lanarkshire Health Board [2015]).

Thus the term *Health Care Professionals (HCPs)* will be used in this chapter when considering professional responsibilities.

The application of principles can be a useful means of helping us to focus on the patient and can be helpful in avoiding self-interest. The Four Principles approach of Beauchamp and Childress (2019) has become well known as a tool to help HCPs in making decisions. The principles to be taken into account are: autonomy, beneficence, non-maleficence and justice. The first of these principles, autonomy, means being able to make one's own decisions and to have these decisions respected by HCPs. To be beneficent is to do good and when caring for a patient with capacity, respecting the exercise of their autonomy is increasingly regarded as the highest good we can provide. As already noted, ethics is about what we do and as HCPs we have a duty to be clinically competent, and especially when caring for patients without capacity, we are expected to uphold their best interests. Patients expect to benefit from our care.

Non-maleficence is what might be described as the bottom line, it is the standard beneath which we must not fall because if we do the patient may suffer harm. It is at this point that the courts may become involved if a patient or their family argues they have been harmed as a result of a failure in acceptable standards.

Activity 11.1

Before the chapter proceeds, take some time to reflect on the four principles and examples from your own practice when you or others have been challenged in upholding them.

A claim in negligence can be made if a patient or others on their behalf can show that they suffered harm as result of our failure to meet an acceptable professional standard. The cases discussed below show how the standards the law expects us to meet in relation to consent must be met to uphold the rights of patients and to avoid a claim of negligence.

The NHS constitution (Department of Health, 2015) says:

> You have the right to accept or refuse treatment that is offered to you, and not to be given any physical examination or treatment unless you have given valid consent. If you do not have the capacity to do so, consent must be obtained from a person legally able to act on your behalf, or the treatment must be in your best interests.

This reflects the legal position, understanding of which is crucial for the giving of holistic care. In England and Wales the Mental Capacity Act 2005 provides the legal framework governing consent. In Scotland this is provided by the Adults with Incapacity Act (Scotland) 2000. Both of these Acts are accompanied by Codes of Practice, which are available for consultation online. In Scotland this is provided by the Adults with Incapacity Act (Scotland) 2000. In Northern Ireland this is provided by The Mental Capacity Act (NI) 2016. These Acts are accompanied by Codes of Practice which are available for consultation online.

THE MENTAL CAPACITY ACT (MCA)

The MCA 2005 begins with the statement of five principles.

Principles of the MCA

The following principles apply for the purposes of this Act:

- A person must be assumed to have capacity unless it is established that he lacks capacity.
- A person is not to be treated as unable to make a decision unless all practicable steps to help him to do so have been taken without success.
- A person is not to be treated as unable to make a decision merely because he makes an unwise decision.
- An act done, or decision made, under this Act for or on behalf of a person who lacks capacity must be done, or made, in his best interests.
- Before the act is done, or the decision is made, regard must be had to whether the purpose for which it is needed can be as effectively achieved in a way that is less restrictive of the person's rights and freedom of action.

(Mental Capacity Act 2005)

The use of the word 'must' in the first principle tells us that this is considered essential. 'The right to decide whether or not to consent to medical treatment is one of the most important rights guaranteed by law' (Heart of England NHS Foundation Trust v JB [2014]). The judgement continues:

… anyone capable of making decisions has an absolute right to accept or refuse medical treatment, regardless of the wisdom or consequences of the decision. The decision does not have to be justified to anyone. In the absence of consent any invasion of the body will be a criminal assault. The fact that the intervention is well-meaning or therapeutic makes no difference.

This is a clear statement of the significance of Sec.1(2) and (4) of the MCA's principles and of the potential consequences for the HCP of being charged with criminal assault if those requirements are ignored.

The HCP will of course encounter patients whose capacity is in doubt. The MCA 2005 states:

People who lack capacity

1) For the purposes of this Act, a person lacks capacity in relation to a matter if at the material time he is unable to make a decision for himself in relation to the matter because of an impairment of, or a disturbance in the functioning of, the mind or brain.

Examples of impairment could be a learning disability, dementia or permanent brain injury. Disturbances in the functioning of the mind or brain can arise from, for example, hypoxia, hypoglycaemia, pyrexia, being under the influence of drugs such as opiates, both prescribed and recreational, and being drunk. A disturbance can usually be resolved but impairment cannot. If it is decided that there is an impairment or disturbance then the professionals need to consider the following:

Is the impairment or disturbance sufficient that the person lacks the capacity to make a particular decision?

This means that a person has to have the capacity specific to the decision that has to be made. The level of capacity needed will depend upon the seriousness of the decision. Someone may therefore be able to make decisions about whether or not to have the winter flu vaccine but not about whether or not to have an operation. This also means that because some individuals lack full capacity their rights to make choices and decisions about their lives cannot be ignored or over-ridden.

Furthermore:

A lack of capacity cannot be established merely by reference to:

a person's age or appearance, or

a condition of his, or an aspect of his behaviour, which might lead others to make unjustified assumptions about his capacity.

(Mental Capacity Act 2005)

The importance of following the spirit of the MCA 2005 in these matters was explored in *Kings College NHS Foundation Trust v C and V* [2015]. C was a woman who in the words of the judge: 'is a person to whom the epithet "conventional"' will never be applied'. As a result of a failed suicide attempt, she had sustained serious renal damage and now required dialysis to maintain her life. She refused this in the knowledge that it would bring about her death. The trust argued that she lacked the capacity to make that decision. The judge began his analysis of the facts by stating:

1.   ... determination of capacity under Part I of the Mental Capacity Act 2005 is always 'decision specific' having regard to the clear structure provided by sections 1 to 3 of the Act ... Thus capacity is required to be assessed in relation to the specific decision at the time the decision needs to be made and not to a person's capacity to make decisions generally.
2.   *... a person is not to be treated as unable to make a decision merely because he or she makes a decision that is unwise.*

It is important in this regard to recall the words of Peter Jackson J in Heart of England NHS Foundation Trust v JB [2014] EWHC 342 (COP) at [7]:

The temptation to base a judgment of a person's capacity upon whether they seem to have made a good or bad decision, and in particular on whether they have accepted or rejected medical advice, is absolutely to be avoided. That would be to put the cart before the horse or, expressed another way, to allow the tail of welfare to wag the dog of capacity. Any tendency in this direction risks infringing the rights of that group of persons who, though vulnerable, are capable of making their own decisions. Many who suffer from mental illness are well able to make decisions about their medical treatment, and it is important not to make unjustified assumptions to the contrary.

The final decision of the judge was that C did have the capacity to make that particular decision but he also said there was nothing to prevent the clinicians continuing to offer the treatment. In citing Peter Jackson J's previous judgement, which has been mentioned earlier in this chapter, McDonald J demonstrated the importance accorded to precedence in English law, i.e. a judge will always look to previous cases with similar facts when making a judgement.

The reason that so much emphasis is placed on capacity is because the patient is being asked to make a decision that may have serious consequences. It is recognised that in order to make a decision information is needed. Section 3 of the MCA states that an individual must be able:

a. To understand the information relevant to the decision.
b. To retain that information.
c. To use or weigh that information as part of the process of making the decision.
d. To communicate his decision (whether by talking, using sign language or any other means).

(Mental Capacity Act 2005)

These standards were established by case law decided before the establishment of the MCA in 2005. Their significance was further developed in Montgomery v Lanarkshire Health Board [2015]. Nadine Montgomery gave birth to a baby boy on 1 October 1999. As a result of complications arising from shoulder dystocia during the delivery, the baby was born with severe disabilities. Antenatally, the risk of shoulder dystocia had been assessed in the order of 9–10%, as Mrs Montgomery was diabetic. The doctor did not discuss the risk of shoulder dystocia or counsel the mother in relation to the option of a planned caesarean section. The view was that the risk of serious injury from shoulder dystocia was small at less than 1% and that if advised/warned a caesarean would have been chosen, when that would not have been in her best interest (in the opinion of the clinicians). The judges held that it would be a mistake to view patients as uninformed, incapable of understanding medical matters, or wholly dependent on information from doctors. It was favourably noted that this was reflected in the GMC's guidance, *Decision making and consent* (2020). Given the Supreme Court's approval of this guidance it is worth all HCPs acquainting themselves with its contents. This in turn can lead to better multidisciplinary team working and thus better patient care.

The judgement also showed an increasing consciousness of fundamental values such as self-determination. Lords Kerr and Reed reasoned that adults of sound mind were entitled to decide which of the available treatments to undergo, and the consent of those adults must be obtained before treatment interfering with their bodily integrity is undertaken. The HCP is under a duty to take reasonable care to ensure that the patient is aware of any material risks involved in proposed treatment, and of reasonable alternatives. A risk was 'material' if a reasonable person in the patient's position would be likely to attach significance to it, or if the HCP was or should reasonably be aware that their patient would be likely to attach significance to it. Three further points emerged. First, assessing the significance of a risk is fact-sensitive, cannot be reduced to percentages and must also be sensitive to the characteristics of the patient. In short a 'one size fits all' explanation is not acceptable. It is the responsibility of HCPs to adapt their explanations to the individual. This will be achieved by observing the second point: in order to advise, the HCP must engage in dialogue with the patient. Dialogue entails having a two way conversation:

> ... the aim of which is to ensure that the patient understands the seriousness of her condition, and the anticipated benefits and risks of the proposed treatment and any reasonable alternatives, so that she is then in a position to make an informed decision. This role will only be performed effectively if the information provided is comprehensible. The doctor's duty is not therefore fulfilled by bombarding the patient with technical information which she cannot reasonably be expected to grasp, let alone by routinely demanding her signature on a consent form (Montgomery v Lanarkshire Health Board 2015).

Again, stress is placed on the requirement that explanations are provided in the sort of language that the patient will understand. It is also clear that a signed consent form alone does not constitute evidence that legally valid consent has been obtained.

Third, the therapeutic exception is limited and should not be abused. The therapeutic exception means that information can be withheld from the patient if it is thought that its disclosure would be seriously detrimental to the patient's health. If this approach were to be adopted in relation to the care of a patient it would be advisable to take the decision following an MDT discussion with the reasoning clearly recorded in writing.

In the light of the above, it should come as no surprise that Mrs Montgomery won her case.

In Thefaut v Johnston [2017] the court had to consider a claim in relation to elective surgery both in terms of the information provided prior to consent being given and the level of competence of the actual procedure. The judge ruled that the operation had been carried out to an acceptable standard but that Mrs Thefaut would not have agreed to have the operation had she been provided with a more accurate estimate of success.

There had to be 'adequate time and space' for there to have been a reasonable dialogue and, following from Montgomery v Lanarkshire Health Board [2015] the need for clear and accurate patient focused information to be provided by the HCP in order for the patient to make a properly informed decision was reiterated.

The patient's informed consent means little if it is then not properly documented. While a signed consent form may assist in showing that the consent process has been initiated, it may only pay lip service to informed consent. The judgements in both Montgomery (2015) and Thefaut (2017) warn against the over-reliance on signed consent forms. A full record of discussions and the information provided needs to be made in the patient's medical records. Without this HCPs cannot rely on stating their usual or standard practice to explain what information the patient might have been given.

There are times when it appears that patients' refusal of treatment is so heavily influenced by outside factors that it can no longer be considered their independent decision. Such a situation arose in the case of Re T (adult: refusal of medical treatment) [1992]. T was injured in a car accident when she was 34 weeks pregnant. After speaking to her mother who was a Jehovah's Witness, T repeatedly refused a blood transfusion, despite this being seen as essential to save her life. T said that although she was no longer a Jehovah's Witness herself, she still retained some of the beliefs. The refusal was challenged on the grounds that her mother's influence was so overbearing that it vitiated T's ability to make her own decision.

Overriding T's refusal, the Court said that although every adult had the right and capacity to decide whether to accept medical treatment, even if a refusal might risk permanent injury or even lead to premature death, and regardless of whether the reasons for the refusal were rational or irrational, unknown or even non-existent, if a patient's capacity to make a decision had been overborne by the undue influence of others, it was the duty of the doctors to treat her/him in whatever way they considered, in the exercise of their clinical judgement, to be in her/his best interests.

In NHS Trust v T [2004] a patient with a history of self-harming leading to dangerously low haemoglobin levels refused a transfusion. She knew her refusal might cause her death; nevertheless she believed that her blood was evil and that the healthy blood given her in a transfusion became contaminated and thus increased the volume of evil blood in her body and 'likewise the danger of my committing acts of evil'. The court ruled that she was unable to use and weigh the relevant information, and thus the competing factors, in the process of arriving at her decision to refuse a transfusion. Thus her refusal was considered invalid and the doctors could proceed in her best interests.

While the MCA lays great stress on the importance of respecting and upholding the rights of patients with capacity to make their own decisions, it also recognises in Sections 1(5) and (6) that not all adults have capacity and that decisions will have to be made on their behalf. There are several mechanisms by which this can be done lawfully. The most important of these is an advance directive. The requirements for these are set out in Sections 24, 25 and 26 of the MCA. To be lawful an advance directive has to be valid and applicable. Validity means that it was drawn up by a person over the age of 18 who had capacity at the time of making it. Applicability means that it applies to the treatment needed at the time it comes into use (Sec. 26(1) MCA). An advance decision only comes into force when a patient has lost capacity. It can only be used to refuse treatment, e.g. to refuse ventilation but not to demand it. However, when decisions are being made about treatment it will be a factor to consider if a patient has said that s/he would want a particular treatment if it was considered in her/his best interests. If the directive states that the patient refuses lifesaving treatment then it must be in writing, signed and witnessed (Sec. 25 MCA). It is not possible to ask for anything unlawful, e.g. a lethal injection. Assisting a suicide remains unlawful throughout the UK (Suicide Act 1961). One of the most important issues to be considered when devising an advance directive is the difficulty of predicting the future. An individual may have seen members of the family suffering from cancer and draw up a directive accordingly but then suffer from a stroke. It is also difficult to predict what advances in the treatment of a disease will be made and thus what the prognosis will be. If a patient has an advance directive it will be useful if it is reviewed regularly in the light of any developments so that it is a true reflection of the patient's current wishes. A valid advance decision to refuse treatment is legally binding on those providing care. It is therefore very important that all appropriate checks are made as to the existence of such a document. In NHS Cumbria CCG v Rushton [2018], Mrs Rushton had made an advance decision to refuse all life sustaining measures in the event of a collapse. After suffering a severe brain injury her life was sustained from December 2015 until December 2018 because in the words of the judge: 'It perhaps requires to be said, though in my view it should be regarded as axiomatic, that the medical profession must give these advanced decisions the utmost care, attention and scrutiny. I am confident the profession does but I regret to say that I do not think sufficient care and scrutiny took place here'.

If there is no advance directive then the next most important means of determining a patient's wishes is through someone who has a Lasting Power of Attorney. This is set up by someone, known as the donor, who is over the age of 18 and while they have capacity. There are two types of Lasting Power of Attorney:

- Health and welfare
- Property and financial affairs

An individual can make one or both. The person or persons given the Lasting Power of Attorney are attorney(s). The donor chooses their attorney(s), who can be anyone they want, and fills in the forms. These can be obtained from the Office of the Public Guardian online or through the post. They must be signed by the donor and witnessed and then registered with the Office of the Public Guardian. Unless the forms are registered, the attorney(s) has no legal standing when decisions have to be made. The sort of decisions that someone with a health and welfare Lasting Power of Attorney can make include:

- The donor's daily routine (e.g. washing, dressing, eating)
- Medical care
- Moving into a care home
- Life-sustaining treatment

It can only be used when the donor is unable to make their own decisions. The HCP will therefore need to check that the attorney is registered with the Office of the Public Guardian as relatives may not understand the need for this. If there is more than one attorney then the forms will stipulate if each attorney can act individually or if they must make decisions jointly. A person with capacity may also end a Lasting Power of Attorney and this must be registered with the Office of the Public Guardian and the attorney(s) informed.

If a patient who lacks capacity has no advance directive or someone with a Lasting Power of Attorney, a Deputy of the Court of Protection may make decisions on the patient's behalf. This will be someone, usually family or a close friend, who has applied to the court to be made a deputy in order to act as a health and social welfare deputy on behalf of an individual who does not have capacity and where there is no other provision made.

If none of the above are in place then it is the responsibility of the HCPs to act in the patient's best interests when deciding on any care or treatment to be given. The Mental Capacity Act 2005 gives some guidance on the factors that should be considered when trying to work out what is in a patient's best interests. These are set out in Section 4(6) of the act as follows:

> In determining for the purposes of this Act what is in a person's best interests, the person making the determination must consider so far as is reasonably ascertainable:
>
> a. the person's past and present wishes and feelings (and, in particular,
>
>   any relevant written statement made by him when he had capacity)
>
> b. the beliefs and values that would be likely to influence his decision if he had capacity, and
>
> c. the other factors that he would be likely to consider if he were able to do so.

The wording of the Act means that while an individual's wishes etc. need to be considered, this does not mean that they will necessarily determine what happens. The doctor will make the final decision about what constitutes 'best interests' unless the courts intervene. In Aintree University Hospitals NHS Foundation Trust v James [2013] Lady Hale provided an analysis of the requirements of Sec. 4 of the MCA:

> The most that can be said, therefore, is that in considering the best interests of this particular patient at this particular time, decision-makers must look at his welfare in the widest sense, not just medical but social and psychological; they must consider the nature of the medical treatment in question, what it involves and its prospects of success; they must consider what the outcome of that treatment for the patient is likely to be; they must try and put themselves in the place of the individual patient and ask what his attitude to the treatment is or would be likely to be; and they must consult others who are looking after him or interested in his welfare, in particular for their view of what his attitude would be.

This statement shows the importance the court places on ensuring that the focus of attention should be the patient and that best interests is not solely a matter of the medical treatment under consideration but the necessity of considering the patient in the context of their beliefs and values. It also means that the people most closely involved in the patient's life must be consulted about their views concerning his or her likely wishes in the context in which they now find themselves.

The judgement also approached the issue of making decisions about the continuation or withdrawal of treatment from a patient who lacks capacity. Lady Hale states that while: 'the starting point is a strong presumption that it is in a person's best interests to stay alive … this is not absolute. There are cases where it will not be in a patient's best interests to receive life-sustaining treatment'.

In making such decisions:

> the fundamental question is whether it is lawful to give the treatment, not whether it is lawful to withhold it. Hence the focus is on whether it is in the patient's best interests to give the treatment, rather than on whether it is in his best interests to withhold or withdraw it. If the treatment is not in his best interests, the court will not be able to give its consent on his behalf and it will follow that it will be lawful to withhold or withdraw it. Indeed, it will follow that it will not be lawful to give it. It also follows that (provided of course that they have acted reasonably and without negligence) the clinical team will not be in breach of any duty towards the patient if they withhold or withdraw it.

> (Aintree University Hospitals NHS Foundation Trust v James [2013] UKSC 67)

Many of the cases that come before the courts which involve decisions about care and treatment for severely ill or disabled patients who lack capacity involve withdrawing Clinically Assisted Nutrition and Hydration (CAHN) from patients in Prolonged Disorders of Consciousness (PDOC), which is the term now used to embrace both Persistent Vegetative State (PVS) and Minimally Conscious State (MCS) in such cases. In An NHS Trust v Y [2018] it was ruled that if the provisions of the MCA are followed and the relevant guidance observed, and if there is agreement upon what is in the best interests of the patient, the patient may be treated in accordance with that agreement without application to the court. This means that family and professionals need to be in agreement. If this cannot be achieved then the case will need to be referred to the courts.

Activity 11.2

Download the Decisions Relating to Cardiopulmonary Resuscitation document here: www.resus.org.uk/library/publications/publication-decisions-relating-cardiopulmonary.

Read the 'Main messages' of the document before returning to the chapter. Given the very serious nature of the decisions being made, time to return to consider the whole document should be made.

Some of the most difficult discussions within acute care involve whether or not to attempt resuscitation. R (Tracey) v Cambridge University Hospitals NHS Foundation Trust & Ors [2014] clarifies what is expected of the HCP in relation to a patient who has capacity. These are:

> Since a DNACPR decision is one which will potentially deprive the patient of life-saving treatment, there should be a presumption in favour of patient involvement. There needs to be convincing reasons not to involve the patient.

> It is inappropriate to involve the patient in the process if the clinician considers that to do so is likely to cause her to suffer physical or psychological harm. Merely causing distress, however, would not be sufficient to obviate the need to involve the patient.

> Where the clinician's decision is that attempting CPR is futile, there is an obligation to tell the patient that this is the decision. The patient may then be able to seek a second opinion (although if the patient's multidisciplinary team all agree that attempting CPR would be futile, the team is not obliged to arrange for a further opinion).

In the case of Winspear v City Hospitals Sunderland NHS Foundation Trust [2015], the court dealt with the rights of patients who lack capacity and the implementation of Do Not Attempt Cardiopulmonary Resuscitation (DNAR) orders. Carl Winspear had cerebral palsy and other severe physical disabilities. He lacked capacity under the MCA 2005 in respect of medical treatment. The decision was taken to put in place a DNAR order in his notes in the very early hours of the morning without consultation with his mother, although the clinician intended to discuss the matter with her at a more convenient time of the day. When his mother learnt of it nine hours later she objected and the order was withdrawn. Carl died later that day.

The judge ruled that the core principles of prior discussion apply equally in all situations regardless of mental capacity. Where a patient lacks the requisite capacity, Section 4(7) MCA encompasses the procedural obligations to consult. This obligation can only be waived in situations where it is truly impracticable or inappropriate to hold such a discussion. The judge held that making a phone call at 3 am might be inconvenient but it was not impracticable. Thus the clinician had failed to meet the requirements of Section 4(7).

This means that good communication skills will be essential in order to initiate such conversations in a tactful and sensitive manner. Patients with capacity are of course free to refuse to engage in the discussion and should not be 'badgered' – the term is used by the family of Mrs Tracey – into doing so. Families and carers will also need to be consulted when considering the best interests of those who lack capacity.

There will inevitably be many occasions in the care of acutely ill patients when the focus of care has to move from restoration to palliation.

PALLIATIVE AND END OF LIFE CARE

The World Health Organisation (2012) defines palliative care as:

> an approach that improves the quality of life of patients and their families facing the problem associated with life-threatening illness, through the prevention and relief of suffering by means of early identification and impeccable assessment and treatment of pain and other problems, physical, psychosocial and spiritual.

Palliative care, prior to the publication of the End of Life Care Strategy (2008), was predominantly associated with terminal cancer diagnosis and hospice care and since then, has been applicable to all patients with a life limiting illness in any care setting. The *Ambitions for palliative and end of life care* (National Palliative and End of Life Care Partnership May, 2021) builds on the strategy with the following ambitions:

- Each person is seen as an individual.
- Each person gets access to care.
- Maximising comfort and wellbeing.
- Care is coordinated.
- All staff are prepared to care.
- Each community is prepared to help.

The UK was the first country to have a strategy that promoted high quality end of life care for all adults, and in 2015 the UK was ranked as having the best palliative care in the world. The strategy highlighted that all care settings should be delivering good quality end of life care as not all patients die in a hospice, which is seen as the gold standard. In fact in 2016 only 5.7% of deaths occurred in a hospice, 21.8% in a care home, 23.5% at home and 46.9% of people died in a hospital (Public Health England, 2018). Age is a factor in where a person dies with over half of deaths of those aged 75–84 occurring in hospital and 36.7% of those aged over 85 were in a care home. Demographic changes to the population indicate that the number of deaths will be higher than the number of births for the first time in 2030 and where people die will also change with more dying in institutional care or in hospitals (Gomes & Higginson, 2008).

Activity 11.3

Consider why it is difficult to discuss end of life care with patients. You may like to conduct a literature search in this area.

These changes mean that there is a need to have more conversations with more people who are admitted to hospital and care facilities about end of life care so that interventional care is not always seen as the default position for everyone. This includes those patients in acute care settings and the recent international COVID-19 pandemic has highlighted the importance of integrating a palliative non-maleficent approach to care.

The actual numbers of death from COVID-19 are as yet to be fully reported, but the UK death rate at the time of writing (April 2021) was over 120,000 and this has required HCPs to adapt quickly to how they approach the subject of treatment options especially in emergency situations, and the withholding of non-beneficial treatments from very sick patients, when ordinarily these options would be offered due to not wanting to give up trying to 'save' someone.

Emergency care plans (ECPs) allow clinicians to discuss and record patients' preferences in advance related to all care and treatment options in emergency situations, which is tailored to the individual and can apply to a sudden acute illness, cardiac or respiratory arrest or a deterioration of a long term condition (Pitcher et al., 2017). The Resuscitation Council UK (2020) has developed a process for recording these ECPs – Recommended Summary Plan for Emergency Care and Treatment (ReSPECT). The process is created by undertaking a conversation between a person and one or more HCP.

A ReSPECT conversation follows the ReSPECT process by:

1. Discussing and reaching a shared understanding of the person's current state of health and how it may change in the foreseeable future.
2. Identifying the person's preferences for and goals of care in the event of a future emergency.
3. Using that to record an agreed focus of care as being more towards life-sustaining treatments or more towards prioritising comfort rather than efforts to sustain life.
4. Making and recording shared decisions about specific types of care and realistic treatment that they would want considered, or that they would not want, and explaining sensitively advance decisions about treatments that clearly would not work in their situation.
5. Making and recording a shared decision about whether or not CPR is recommended.

(Resuscitation Council UK, 2020)

Acute and community care providers are able to implement the ReSPECT process so that the ECP can be recognised across all care providers in a location. The documents are different to ADRT as they are not legally binding and they are used as part of the advance care planning process. They can be written when a person is fit and healthy and can record wishes in case of an unexpected emergency in the future at their request. ECP discussions do not just apply to patients in hospital, but those who are admitted to care homes, or in attendance at clinics in primary and secondary care for those who have complex or long term medical needs. Coronavirus has increased the number of people making enquiries about treatment decisions related to the pandemic but also on advance decisions (Compassion in Dying, 2020), with the organisation developing specific resources for Coronavirus and the treatments available and the option to register advance decisions online. Further clarification on conversations related to Coronavirus during the ReSPECT process was also made in April 2020 (Resuscitation Council UK, 2020) to alleviate patient fears that blanket decisions on resuscitation would be made on patients due to age or pre-existing diseases.

It is of course easier to have a conversation about emergency care with a person who knows what they want in an emergency or end of life situation, but not all HCPs feel confident in having the conversation or broaching the subject; however patients do expect the HCP to take the lead.

Communication and advance planning

Communication is a key part of palliative and end of life care; honest open conversations happen on a day to day basis. However this is not the same for all HCPs especially those working in acute care, as discussed by Atul Gawande, an American surgeon, who explains that he has had to learn a different approach to conversations when talking to patients about treatment options (2014). He advocates enabling wellbeing rather than striving for survival, and to do this conversations are key to have, but not necessarily starting with the options available, but instead discussing what is important to the person now and in the future. For example, a discussion with a 94 year old lady living independently when asked about her wishes to go to hospital, should she have another exacerbation of her heart failure, refused, as her greatest pleasure was being at home with her dog and being able to see him play in the garden with her great grandson. This was good for her wellbeing and whilst acknowledging that hospital treatment might make her better, she knew her time was precious. This conversation led to the lady making an advance decision to refuse treatment, which she discussed with her family and GP so that the next time she became less well she was cared for at home as per her wishes. Any type of advance care planning, discussions or documentation can improve end of life care experience for patients as well as the experience of the bereaved (Levoy et al., 2020; NICE, 2018).

The Serious Illness Care Programme UK (n.d.) have carried out research into how HCPs can use language and open questions to improve patient experience and for them to express their values as well as what is important to them when facing a serious illness or a worsening of condition. The programme is building on the work carried out by Atul Gawande in the USA, which has demonstrated that 86% of patients benefit from meaningful conversations, and 90% of clinicians have adopted the approach into their own practice. By using the serious illness conversation guide, the language used for a discussion is very different (see Table 11.1).

Table 11.1 The serious illness conversation guide

Understanding	What is your understanding now of where you are with your illness?
Information preferences	How much information about what is likely to be ahead with your illness would you like from me?
Prognosis	Share prognosis, tailored to information preferences.
Goals	If your health situation worsens, what are your most important goals?
Fears/worries	What are your biggest fears and worries about the future with your health?
Function	What abilities are so critical to your life that you can't imagine living without them?
Trade-offs	If you became sicker, how much are you willing to go through for the possibility of gaining more time?
Family	How much does your family know about your priorities and wishes?

This approach makes the conversation less about treatment options and DNACPR but concentrates on the reality of having a serious illness from which the person may not recover, and addresses the issues that are important to them. Very often this does not concern their treatment but their family, pets, upcoming events, holidays, and opportunities to fulfil lifetime wishes. Having this conversation is keeping with the palliative care philosophy of living until you die, and as shown, can really improve the experience of end of life care not just for patients, but their loved ones and the staff caring for them.

SUMMARY

This chapter has focused on legal and ethical perspectives in acute care, withdrawal of treatment, do not attempt resuscitation orders, palliative and end of life care and the non-technical skills required to deliver compassionate care.

REFERENCES

Aintree University Hospitals NHS Foundation Trust v James [2013] UKSC 67.

An NHS Trust v Y (Intensive Care Society & Ors intervening) [2018] UKSC 46.

Beauchamp, T.L. & Childress, J.F. (2019) *Principles of Biomedical Ethics*. New York: Oxford University Press.

Compassion in Dying (2020) *Living wills skyrocket in light of coronavirus* [online]. Available at: https://compassionindying.org.uk/living-wills-skyrocket-in-light-of-coronavirus/ (accessed 13 February 2022).

Crisp, R. (Ed.) (2014) *Aristotle: Nicomachean Ethics*. Cambridge: Cambridge University Press.

Cummings, J. & Bennett, V. (2012) *Compassion in Practice: Nursing, Midwifery and Care Staff: our Vision and Strategy*, Gateway reference 18479. London: Department of Health.

Department of Health (2015) *The NHS Constitution for England*, updated 2021. Available from: www.gov.uk/government/publications/the-nhs-constitution-for-england/the-nhs-constitution-for-england (accessed 31 January 2022).

Gawande, A. (2007) *Better: A Surgeon's Notes on Performance*. New York: Macmillan.

Gawande, A. (2014) *Being Mortal*. London: Profile Books Limited.

General Medical Council (GMC) (2020) *Decision making and consent*. Available at: https://www.gmc-uk.org/-/media/documents/gmc-guidance-for-doctors---decision-making-and-consent-english_pdf-84191055.pdf (accessed 13 February 2022).

Gomes, B. & Higginson, I. (2008) Where people die (1974–2030): Past trends, future projections and implications for care. *Palliative Medicine*, 22 (1), 33–41.

Heart of England NHS Foundation Trust v JB [2014] EWHC 342 (COP).

Kings College NHS Foundation Trust v C and V [2015] EWCOP 80.

Levoy, K., Buck, H. & Behar-Zusman (2020) The impact of varying levels of advance care planning engagement on perceptions of the end of life experience among caregivers of deceased patients with cancer. *American Journal of Hospice and Palliative Medicine*, 37 (12). doi: 10.1177/1049909120917899.

Mental Capacity Act 2005 (c.9). Available at: https://www.legislation.gov.uk/ukpga/2005/9/contents (accessed 5 May 2022).

Montgomery v Lanarkshire Health Board [2015] UKSC 1.

National Palliative and End of Life Care Partnership (2021) *Ambitions for palliative and end of life care*. Available at: www.england.nhs.uk/wp-content/uploads/sites/48/2021/10/FINAL_Ambiti onsforPalliativeandEndofLifeCare_2nd_edition.pdf (accessed 31 January 2022).

NHS Cumbria CCG v Rushton [2018] EWCOP 41.

NHS Trust v T [2004] EWHC 1279.

NICE (2018) *Advance care planning*, NG94. Available at: www.nice.org.uk/guidance/ng94/evidence/15.advance-care-planning-pdf-172397464602 (accessed 31 January 2022).

Nursing and Midwifery Council (NMC) (2018) *The Code: Professional Standards of Practice and Behaviour for Nurses and Midwives*. London: NMC.

Pitcher, D., Fritz, D., Wang, M. & Spiller, J. (2017) Emergency and resuscitation plans. *BMJ*, 356, 876.

Public Health England (2018) *Palliative and end of life care profiles*. Available at: https://fingertips.phe.org.uk/profile/end-of-life (accessed 31 January 2022).

R (Tracey) v Cambridge University Hospitals NHS Foundation Trust & Ors [2014] EWCA Civ 822.

R v. Instan (1893) 1 QB 450.

Re T (adult: refusal of medical treatment) [1992] 4 All ER 649 (CA).

Resuscitation Council UK (2020) *ReSPECT*. Available at: www.resus.org.uk/respect (accessed 31 January 2022).

Serious Illness Care Programme UK (n.d.) *Serious Illness Care Programme UK*. Available at: https://betterconversations.org.uk/ (accessed 31 January 2022).

The World Health Organisation (2012) *Palliative care*. Available at: www.who.int/cancer/palliative/definition/en/ (accessed 31 January 2022).

Thefaut v. Johnston [2017] EWHC 497 QB.

Winspear v City Hospitals Sunderland NHS Foundation Trust [2015] EWHC 3250 (QB).

INDEX

NOTE: page numbers in *italic* type refer to figures and tables.

Ingram Content Group UK Ltd.
Milton Keynes UK
UKHW051942280423
420951UK00004B/34